DATE DUE

MAY 1 1 2007		
NOV 3 0 2009		
MAR 2 9 2016		
MAY 0 4 2017		
DISCARDED		

The

PURPLE
GUIDE

DEVELOPING YOUR CLINICAL DENTAL HYGIENE CAREER

Shirley Gutkowski, RDH, BSDH
Amy Nieves, RDH

Exploring Transitions
Sun Prairie, WI

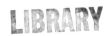
Published by Exploring Transitions
P.O. Box 194
Sun Prairie, WI 53590

Publisher's Cataloguing-in-Publication Data
Gutkowski, Shirley.

The purple guide : developing your clinical dental hygiene career/Shirley Gutkowski, Amy Nieves. – Sun Prairie, WI : Exploring Transitions, 2004.

p. ; cm.
Includes index.
ISBN: 0-9749478-0-6

1. Dental hygiene–Vocational guidance. 2. Career development. 3. Dental hygienists. I. Nieves, Amy. II. Title.

RK60.5 .G88 2004   2004104300
617.6/01/023--dc22   0406

Book production and coordination by Jenkins Group, Inc.
www.bookpublishing.com
Interior design by Barbara Hodge
Cover design by Kelli Leader

Printed in the United States of America
08 07 06 05 04 • 5 4 3 2 1

Contents

Why This Book?

A my Nieves and I decided to write this book together because we were both scared to death after we graduated from our respective dental hygiene programs. We still had so many questions at graduation. It took me forever to figure some things out. Working without another hygienist to bounce things off was very difficult.

With the introduction of the Internet, the questions got easier to answer, and isolation was overcome. It was easier to find out new things, progress was suddenly moving at a pace so fast that it sometimes left you gasping for air.

Amy and I first learned of each other on the Internet in 1999. That year, she invited me to join an online discussion group she had started. Over the years, it became increasingly apparent that this group of hygienists had all the same issues that we did. New graduates all had the same questions, and most felt unprepared to work with the complexities of the real world.

As Amy and I got to know each other better through the group over the Internet, we became friends. We had a long-distance relationship: She lived in New Jersey and I lived in Wisconsin. We met each other for the first time in 2000 as members of the 3M ESPE Dental Hygiene Advisory Panel. We discussed the issues that are universal in the conversations on the Internet group. Eventually, I grew serious about writing and became better known in the dental hygiene community through my column in *RDH* magazine. Amy became familiar for her

Internet activities at www.amyrdh.com and the Internet groups that involved dental hygienists and students. We both have monthly columns now in traditional publications that reach tens of thousands of our peers. We knew something was still missing, though. There had to be a way to reach more students, or new graduates, so that they didn't feel so overwhelmed and afraid of what would happen after graduation. We agreed we each had a unique insight into the world of dental hygiene and that a book for this niche was the answer.

We realized that instructors only have a small amount of time to cover all the aspects of real-world dental hygiene. In a program with three to five instructors, there are a finite number of practical working strategies that the instructors have to share with their students. With the Internet list and Amy's Web site, we had thousands of years of practical dental hygiene experience to tap.

The name of the book, *The Purple Guide*, evolved from the color of dentistry, lilac. To illustrate immediately the target audience of this book and to keep the title from sounding like a book on gardening, we decided to use the parent color of lilac, purple.

In the following pages, you'll learn about insurance codes, how to ask for a raise, what questions to ask in an interview, and many other things that you may never have considered before. Dental hygiene is a rewarding career full of wonderful relationships and role modeling opportunities, and it can also bring enormous frustrations. It takes a special person to be a hygienist. What you learned in school is a tiny part of the whole package. This book will help you over the first bumpy stretches on the road to making a difference to patients every 60 minutes.

We hope you'll find this information helpful throughout the beginning of your clinical practice. We invite you to join the Internet group by going to www.amyrdh.com, and click on Join the Email Community button, then learn from others in your profession as we did. Many of the tips in this book are from the dedicated hygienists who post on that site. Welcome to your book.

Shirley Gutkowski

Acknowledgments

We would like to acknowledge the help of the people who had faith in our ability to produce a product that would help thousands of hygienists every day of every year.

Mark Gutkowski

Joe Nieves

Anne M. Durr

Anne Guignon, RDH, MPH
www.ergosonics.com

Beth Thompson, RDH, BS
www.beththompsonrdh.com

Emily Kinsell Berger, RDH, BS
www.emilykinsellberger.com

Dr. Mike Maroon
www.genr8tnext.com

Dr. Steven Wilson

All the hygienists at www.amyrdh.com

1

Preparing for Your New Career

Well, you've done it. You've scrounged up enough Class III and IV patients, and spent more money than you thought you could. You have sacrificed free time and at least three years of full-time working wages. You now have or will soon have a license that allows you to lay your healing hands on a willing, paying patient without benefit of someone looking over your shoulder. No one will recheck your work for a grade. You're responsible for your own work now. Congratulations on finishing the first part of your career path. Ahead of you is a time of change—a time of transition. You are at the drawing board, creating a plan for your professional future. Once you pass your exams, the groundwork is finished. Now the real challenge begins—finding a job. Where to start?

Before you can become successfully employed, you will need to develop and initiate your job search. This chapter will assist you in understanding and following through with four necessary steps of a successful job search.

- Putting "You" into Words
- Where to Work—Location and the Cost of Commuting
- Job Openings—Where to Find Them
- The Job Interview
- Interview Questions to Ask

Putting "You" into Words

A resume must look and sound professional. To quote the older-than-dirt adage: You have to spend money to make money. Here is a short list of things you will need for preparing your resume and conducting your job search:

- Good quality paper and envelopes for your resume (some references suggest using envelopes large enough to allow you to send the resume without folding it)
- A standard spiral notebook in which you can keep a journal of your job search
- Access to a laser printer

A resume is a sales tool. It's the first impression you make on a prospective employer. This little piece of paper is your message to let someone know who you are, what you can deliver, and your what your assets are.

It's a good idea to do a little work before sitting down to write a resume, including doing a self-assessment on paper. Outline your skills and abilities as well as your work experience and extracurricular activities. Assess what classes you enjoyed the most. Which ones drove you crazy? Did you love working with children or the elderly? What turns you on about dental hygiene, and what turns you off? Doing a self-assessment of your strengths and weaknesses will streamline your resume-building process.

You don't need to reinvent the wheel with your resume. There are numerous resources on how to develop one. Using a search engine on the Internet, you can find a multitude of informational sites outlining the resume process. Word processing programs (such as MS Word) have built-in resume templates. The template is a great guide—all you need to do is add the right descriptive words to illustrate who you are to someone who might only have a fraction of a second to get to know you.

You will see several parts in a resume template: Objective, Background, Education, Personal interests, and References.

Depending upon the template that is used, these headings may have other, similar titles. Take some time to consider what should be included under the template headings—it is a good idea to put each heading on a separate piece of paper, and then begin a rough draft for each one. You are actually

Speedy Story
Amy once got a nasty e-mail from someone who thought tootyclnr@aol.com gave the wrong impression of our profession.

just talking about yourself. Let it all hang out. Ask one of your friends to help you if you can't bring yourself to list your strengths.

Here are some more tips:

- All of your contact information should go at the top of your resume.
- Avoid nicknames.
- Use a permanent address.
- Use a permanent telephone number and include the area code.
- If you have an answering machine, record a neutral greeting.
- Include:
  —*key or special skills or competencies*
  —*leadership experience in volunteer organizations*
  —*participation in sports.*
- Add your e-mail address. Many employers will find it useful. (Note: Choose an e-mail address that sounds professional.)
- Include your Web site address only if it reflects your professional ambitions.
- Be specific about the job you want. For example: To work in a progressive general dental practice and help a wide variety of patients keep their teeth a lifetime.
- New graduates without a lot of work experience should list their educational information first. Experienced hygienists can list work experience first.

The Objective tells potential employers the sort of work you expect to provide. Stating your needs or wants in this way will also solidify your ideas and make it less likely that you will settle for an inferior office. This section is one of the most important parts of the resume and one that is usually overlooked. Let the reader of your resume know what type of person you are and what type of job you want. Use key words, often times called buzzwords or jargon, such as:

- recent grad—dental hygienist
- people oriented
- relationship focus
- free thinker
- task oriented
- goal oriented
- multi-task
- periodontal focus
- full-time/part-time
- with benefits/without benefits.

Swift Tip

Add your own buzzwords

This is a good place to let the reader know what type of dental office you're looking for, such as:

- professional
- progressive
- preventive
- large/small office
- multi-location
- private practice
- tells potential employers the sort of work you expect to provide.

A word about references. Always personally speak to everyone you wish to use as a reference, if you cannot speak to them face-to-face, then at least talk with them over the phone. Explain your job search, what type of job you are applying for and why, and tell them that you would like to use them for a reference. If they agree, then it is also a courtesy to let them know to whom you have applied. That

Swift Tips

- *Use good white or off-white paper.*
- *Use 8-1/2- x 11-inch paper.*
- *Use 1" margins. Larger margins are a cheap trick to make something look like more.*
- *Print on only one side of the paper. This is not the time to pinch pennies. Set the printer to print with the best quality.*
- *Use a font size of 12 or 14 points. If this is your very first job, you may want to use the larger font to take up some room on the paper.*
- *Use non-decorative typefaces. Use bold for your name, contact information, and headings.*
- *Choose one font and stick to it. The classics are best, such as Book Antiqua or Times New Roman. If the letters have little ends on them called serifs, they're easier to read than a font without. Arial and Tohoma don't have serifs.*
- *Avoid italics, script, and underlined words.*
- *Do not staple your resume.*
- *If you must mail your resume, put it in a large envelope that matches your paper.*

way your references know who might be calling them. Also, ask people when they can best be reached for a contact.

Following are samples of resumes. Due to space considerations, the font has been sized to fit the page. The font size for your resume should be between 10 and 14. The first resume is the one Amy used immediately after graduation. Notice how it highlights Amy's education by providing it first, then breaking down what she did best at while in college.

Amy M. Nieves, RDH
Street address
City, state, and zip
Phone
E-mail address

Objective

Patient-oriented hygienist seeks to work in a quality office centered on patient's needs and prevention. I'm looking for an office where my skills and education are utilized to benefit your practice growth and success while expanding personal knowledge.

Education

1994—1999   Middlesex County College   Edison, NJ
AAS in Dental Hygiene

- Extensive experience in a clinical setting
- Experience in periodontal screening, treatment, and therapy
- Emphasis on patient education for prevention of oral diseases
- Expanded functions such as sealants, amalgam polishing, oral irrigation, nutritional counseling, plaque control, and radiographs
- Developed great patient skills
- Certificate of Achievement for outstanding academic performance for the academic years 1997-1998 and 1998-1999
- Certificate of Achievement for achieving a GPA of 3.7 and higher on May 21, 1999
- Received the Dental-Search Inc. Recognition Award for efforts in dental hygiene on May 21, 1999
- Maintained dean's list status

Work experience

1988—present   Avalon Avery Apartments   Edison, NJ
Rental Agent

- Worked on weekends as the rental agent. Job entailed helping perspective tenants with renting information and leases, collecting rent payments, and handling maintenance requests. I was in charge of the office on the weekends.

Volunteer experience

Girl Scout leader from 1994-1998

References

Available on request

Accreditations and licenses

Passed National Boards and both sections of the North East Regional Boards. I am awaiting my license, which is expected in July.

This second resume is the one Amy is using now. As you will see, it's updated with all her dental hygiene experience since she graduated. It's two pages long.

Amy M. Nieves, RDH
Street address
City, state, and zip
Phone
E-mail address

Objective

Patient-oriented hygienist seeks to work in a quality office centered on patient's needs and prevention. I'm looking for an office where my skills and education are utilized to benefit your practice growth and success while expanding personal knowledge.

Work experience

April 2002—present   Dr. A   Las Vegas, NV
Dental Hygienist
- Performing prophylaxis, extensive periodontal therapy, use of intraoral camera, patient education, digital radiographs, sealants, local anesthesia, nitrous oxide, EagleSoft software.

January 2001—June 2002   Dr. B   Las Vegas, NV
Dental Hygienist
- Performing prophylaxis, taking radiographs, giving oral hygiene instruction; work schedule is Monday through Thursday.

January 2000—Jan. 2001   Dr. C   Henderson, NV
Dental Hygienist
- Performing prophylaxis, daily scaling and root planings, taking radiographs, giving oral hygiene instruction, maintaining recall system, sealants, use of Dentrix system.

2000—present   A National Dental Hygiene Board Review company
Webmaster
- Responsible for updates to Web site; designed and maintained Web site; part-time position; worked from home.

1999—2000   Dr. D   Somerset, NJ
Dental Hygienist
- Performing prophylaxis, daily scaling and root plannings, taking radiographs, giving oral hygiene instruction, maintaining recall system, sealants, soft tissue management

system, use of Piezo scaler and intra-oral camera, and ordering hygiene supplies.

1988—1999   Avalon Avery Apartments   Highland Park, NJ
Rental Agent
- Part-time rental agent, office manager on weekends; job entailed helping perspective tenants with renting information, and leases, collecting rent payments, and handling maintenance requests; left to pursue dental hygiene career

Education

1994—1999   Middlesex County College   Edison, NJ
AAS in Dental Hygiene
- Extensive experience in a clinical setting; experience in periodontal screening, treatment, and therapy; emphasis on patient education for prevention of oral diseases; expanded functions such as sealants, amalgam polishing, oral irrigation, nutritional counseling, plaque control, and radiographs; developed great patient skills
- Certificate of Achievement for outstanding academic performance for the academic years 1997-1998 and 1998-1999
- Certificate of Achievement for achieving a GPA of 3.7 and higher on May 21, 1999
- Received the Dental-Search Inc. Recognition Award for efforts in dental hygiene on May 21, 1999
- Maintained dean's list status

Licenses

- New Jersey license #XYZ
- Nevada license #XYZ, license to administer local anesthesia and nitrous oxide

Professional memberships & activities

- 1999-present Member of the American Dental Hygienists' Association
- 2000-2003 Secretary Southern Nevada Dental Hygienists' Association (SNDHA)
  2003-2004 Newsletter editor SNDHA
  2000-present Webmaster for the Nevada Dental Hygienists' Association
- Designing and maintaining Web sites
- My own Web site www.amyrdh.com
- http://rdhstudyclub.com
- http://www.amyrdh2.com
- March 2001 cover of *RDH* magazine
- June 2002 cover of *Contemporary Oral Hygiene*

- Interviewed for the ADHA's *Access* magazine.
- Invitation to compile monthly column, "Hygiene Solutions," in *Contemporary Oral Hygiene* evolved from my monitoring the group at YahooGroups on the Internet
- RDH e-mail community with over 1400 worldwide members. (I started this e-mail community in January 1999. Participants include columnists, magazine publishers, CE course presenters, and day-to-day hygienists. This e-mail community has been mentioned in *RDH* magazine and many hygiene seminars across the country.)
- Awarded Honorary Mentor of the Year 2003 by Philips Sonicare and *RDH* magazine
- Key influencer member for *RDH* magazine
- 3M Dental Hygiene Advisory Panel member 2001-present
- Discus Dental Hygiene Panel member October 2002

Volunteer Experience

- Girl Scout leader from 1994-1998.
- Designed and started the New Jersey Dental Hygienists' Association Web site
- Designed and still maintain the Nevada Dental Hygienists' Association Web site

References

Excellent references available upon request

This third resume is one that Amy used when she was looking for temporary work. It's limited to only her work experience. Notice that her license number is included in the Objectives section, proving that she has the education.

Amy M. Nieves, RDH
Street address
City, state, and zip
Phone
E-mail address

Objective—weekly summer work schedule during summer office break

Patient-oriented hygienist seeking summer work schedule—40 hours per week during summer office break—three-week time period (July 2-6, July 23-27, and August 20-24) in a quality office centered on patients' needs and prevention.

Seeking an office environment where my skills and education are utilized to benefit your practice growth and success while expanding personal knowledge. Currently employed full-time, four-day-a-week work schedule with Dr. A's office. (Nevada dental hygiene license number 12345).

Work experience

April 2002—present   Dr. A   Las Vegas, NV
Dental Hygienist
• Performing prophylaxis, extensive periodontal therapy, use of intraoral camera, patient education, digital radiographs, EagleSoft software.

January 2001—June 2002   Dr. B   Las Vegas, NV
Dental Hygienist
• Performing prophylaxis, taking radiographs, giving oral hygiene instruction; work schedule is Monday through Thursday.

2000—January 2001   Dr. C   Henderson, NV
Dental Hygienist
• Performing prophylaxis, daily scaling and root planing, taking radiographs, giving oral hygiene instruction, maintaining recall system, sealants, use of Dentrix system.

2000 -2002   A National Board Review company
Webmaster
• Responsible for updates to Web site; designed and maintained Web site at: www.X.com; part-time position, worked from home.

1999—2000   Dr. D   Somerset, NJ
Dental Hygienist
• Performing prophylaxis, daily scaling and root planing, taking radiographs, giving oral hygiene instruction, maintaining recall

system, sealants, soft tissue management system, use of Piezo
Scaler and intra-oral camera, ordering of hygiene supplies.

1988—1999   Avalon Avery Apartments   Highland Park, NJ

Rental Agent

• Part-time rental agent, office manager on weekends; job
  entailed helping perspective tenants with renting information
  and leases, collecting rent payments, and handling
  maintenance requests.

The easiest way to write a letter of interest/response or cover
letter is called the "T-bar" technique. You simply state in your first
paragraph that you are replying to the prospective employer's
classified ad or job opening. The second paragraph is set up like a
T-bar (see below). The third paragraph is the closing, where you state
your interest in the opening, say that you are looking forward to
hearing from them, and give your contact information—home phone
with answering machine, cell phone, and e-mail address.

Office Requirements	Your Expertise
• licensed dental hygienist • knowledge in "x" procedures	• recent graduate, licensed • proficient in "x" procedures • classes successfully taken in school (list classes)

Your education was built on science, not wordsmithing. Since the
information in your resume is the first impression you'll give, it helps
to use Word Find and a thesaurus to keep from repeating the same
set of words over and over. Most word processing programs come
equipped with a thesaurus. Learn to use it if you haven't already.
After the rough draft of your resume is completed, check to see how
many times you have repeated a word or set of words. It is very
simple to use the thesaurus on the computer or a book to find
several different words that all have the same meaning. Print out your
resume several times and read it with a critical eye. Every time you do
you'll find something to make it better.

Where to Work—Location and the Cost of Commuting

Before you start sending off your resume, you need to decide where you want to work geographically. Figure out how much it will cost you to travel to the office location. Commuting costs figure into the earnings equation. When deciding on a rate of pay—how much you will be earning, per hour, day, or week—you need to calculate how much spendable income you will have after deducting necessary expenses such as commuting costs.

You'll need to review what mode of transportation you will be using to get to work. If you drive, you need to know how much it will cost in time and gasoline for a round trip to work, whether there are road tolls, the roads you will use, and whether you will be commuting in heavy traffic.

If your car is brand new, you will have the benefit of choosing jobs anywhere. The newer your car, the better chance you will have of commuting to work without having engine problems or car maintenance.

Basically speaking, it is best to stay within 15 miles one-way (30 miles round trip) for driving to work. If you will be commuting to

work using public transportation, or using a combination of both your car and public transportation, you can widen the radius to where you work because you won't be driving the entire distance, which can be like work, especially in heavy traffic.

Remember, the amount of time and the distance you travel to work will figure into the equation of how much you need to earn each week. Higher commuting expenses equal lower income. Should you have a choice of two similar jobs, one being 10 miles from home and the other being 20 miles from home, it would be normally better to choose the one closer to home, because the cost of that commute is less in time and money giving you more spendable income for yourself.

Job Openings—Where to Find Them

Now that you have your resume and know the distances you're willing to travel, how do you find job openings? First of all, check with your school. Many schools have career counseling services with current job openings. Some schools incorporate a mentoring system where you can talk with past graduates. They can help you with understanding the industry and possibly with job leads.

Another idea is to check with dental hygienists' associations—national and local groups:

- **National**
  American Dental Hygienists' Association
  444 North Michigan Avenue, Suite 3400
  Chicago, IL 60611
  E-mail: mail@adha.net
  Web: http://www.adha.org

- **Local**

Swift Tip

You can also take the following steps to ensure quality in your resume:

- *Run a spell check on your computer before anyone sees your resume, but don't count on it. There are some words that are spelled correctly, yet are the wrong word for the context. Get a friend (maybe an English major or English instructor) to do a grammar review and proofread. The more eyes that see your resume the less the chance there is that something inappropriate or incorrect will slip though.*

- *Print it out and read it again. It's amazing what stands out once the words are on the paper. To save money, print it on the backside of some other paper, and set your printer options to print in the draft mode.*

- *Printing in a different font will also bring out different aspects and qualities.*

Some local associations can be found through the national Web site, while others can be found by using a search engine on the computer, such as google.com.

Once you decide where you want to work, check out the newspaper classified ads that cover those locations. Other, less traditional

Swift Tip

Distance comes second, of course, if you have options between an office with better quality of care and/or more potential for growth.

sources of information on possible job openings are your friends, suppliers/vendors, employment or temporary agencies, state employment departments, non-dental friends, or dental association newsletters.

Now you will begin to contact dental offices that are looking to hire someone with your qualifications. You can call to see if the job is still open and then schedule an interview by phone, or you can simply mail your resume with an attached letter of interest.

Keep a job journal to keep track of the dates you applied for job openings, what job openings you applied for, and what, if any, follow-up you received from these applications. After the interview, record the date(s), the name of the person/people you met, and the outcome of the interview.

Job Journal—Written Format
- Should you not want to keep your information in a database format, it is a simple process to keep a written journal.
- You can use a spiral notebook, or keep preprinted sheets in a file folder.

Informational data setup:
- Devote a separate page to each job position.
- Make separate headings for each category.

Swift Tip

Sometimes dentists don't post ads in the paper for jobs. It may be worth your time to drop off your resume to offices in your area and ask them to keep it on file for future openings. Do this often.

Job Title: _____
Name of primary contact: _____

Name of Dental Office/Group: _____

Address: _____
City: _____ State: _____ Zip Code: ____
Phone: _____
E-mail: _____ (Person's Name)
Fax: _____

Source:
Newspaper: _____ Date of Ad: _____
Internet _____ Date: _____
Referral: _____ Date: _____
(Name of Person or Agency)

Contact:
Date of First Contact: _____
Phone: _____
Letter/Resume: _____

Result of Contact:
Phone Interview:
      Date: Contact Name: Result: Interview?
                               Phone #:
                               E-mail:

Scheduled Personal Interview:
      Date: Contact Name: Result: 2nd interview?
                               Phone #:   Job Offer
                               E-mail:

Thank-You Responses:
      Date: Contact: Letter/E-mail

Outcome of Interview(s):
      Job Offer
      You Accepted: You Declined: Why? Did not like office
                                       Did not like commute
                                       Pay not right, hours not
                                       right, etc.

Journal   Position: Dental Hygienist

First Response Date to Job Opening	Source	Office or Group Name	Address	Phone#	Email	Fax#	Contact	Date of first interview	Whom did you meet with	Thank you Response Sent	Outcome of Interview
Date *Phone Response* *Letter Response*	*Referral, Internet Ad, Newspaper Ad, Agency*						*To whom did you send your letter of inquiry and resume* *Name title phone/ email/fax*		*Name title phone email fax*	*Name title date sent*	*Your impression great good Their impression* lists points of interest: salary dental office hours benefits
								If you find that your first interviews are telephone interviews you can change this column to be:			
								Date of first phone interview			
								and then add another column for:			
								Date of first personal Interview			

Classified Ads

The classified ads are sometimes difficult to read. What exactly does it mean if there's only a post office box number with no phone number? What does it mean if the phone number is listed and there's no answering machine? There are a number of reasons for this secretive type of advertising. If we give the practice the benefit of the doubt, we could imagine that the current hygienist is not performing to standard. Let's say that the doctor or the office manager has had the final confrontation with this hygienist. It's not unreasonable to place a blind ad so that the hygienist at that office won't find out the dentist is looking for a replacement. Some people could produce a pretty ugly scene if they come upon that knowledge, or they may just stop coming to work. Some people don't know how to act professionally.

Some blind ads are designed to protect the office from its own reputation. If you saw the same phone number in an ad for weeks on end, you'd wonder what's up with that office—and rightly so. Some practices can't hold on to hygienists or other staff members because of the quality of workmanship of the dentist, or the difficulty of working with that dentist or another employee.

Look for those things in the ads that you see every week as you get closer to having your license in hand. Be aware that frequency of an ad is not always a bad thing. If the practice is experiencing rapid growth, such as a growing chain of dental offices, there may be room for many new staff members. It may not be that they find it difficult to hire or retain staff.

The Job Interview

You will need to prepare for an interview as diligently as you did for anything else that has lead up to this section. You'll want to be poised, positive, assertive, and willing to ask questions. Usually you will be sending in your resume along with a letter of interest. You will want to keep track of every job you apply for in your job journal.

Preparing for the Interview

What to wear on your interview? A good business suit always works—women can choose a two-piece ensemble with either a skirt or pants. Neutral colors like navy blue or charcoal gray are good choices. Either color will allow you to wear the same suit and simply change the shirt or blouse. A sensible pair of shoes with closed toes is a must, especially for men. Usually black is the best color for shoes, with a matching purse or briefcase. Why dress up? Remember, you will actually be painting a picture of yourself when you appear for your interview. You want your clothes to say that you're serious about this career, not that you look at it as a means to support your tennis habit. Although your resume is your first impression, the interview is like a second chance at a first impression. A nice outfit with coordinating shoes and purse or briefcase, as well as understated makeup for women, is your future employer's first impression of you. He or she may get this information while watching you get out of the car.

Be sure to have several good copies of your resume to take with you to your interview. You never know when an extra copy will be needed. Also, bring a list of your references and hand them to the interviewer if they ask for it.

The Interview: Points to Remember

Even though you have an appointment for your interview, always call on the day of the appointment to make sure the time still works. There may be an emergency patient, and even dentists can be out sick!

Personal questions concern you—and how you and the job's schedule can work together. What is the regular office/work schedule? Are the hours the same every day, or are they different on some days, such as rotating Saturday hours? On which dates is the office closed, and on which is it open? Some offices have regular holiday schedules; others may close for a week every quarter.

Help to make the interview a two-way conversation. You will be asked questions, feel comfortable in answering these questions, and then ask some of your own. Don't be afraid to ask what the interview schedule is. How many days will they be interviewing? How many people have they or will they be interviewing? Will they be getting back to all candidates or only those they are interested in? They expect these kinds of questions, so don't think you're intruding or being presumptuous.

As the interview comes to a close, let the interviewer know if you are interested in the position. Thank them for their time and tell them that you enjoyed speaking or meeting with them. Ask for the names of everyone you spoke with and always send a thank-you note. This can be done with a formal letter or a simple thank-you card. Few people bother to show this courtesy, and if yours is the only thank-you note the office receives, you'll stand out as a caring, thorough professional.

You will learn something new and helpful from every interview. If you are not successful with one job opening, don't be afraid to ask the prospective employer why. Also, you might learn what type of office you would not like as a workplace. Keep your job journal up to date.

You never know who's going to conduct the interview. It may be the dentist, the office manager, or the resident hygienist. Be polite and poised; sit on the edge of the chair. Even if your first impression of the office is negative, act as if your livelihood depended getting this job. The dental community is very small, and news travels. The worst-looking office may be owned by the most powerful dentist in the tri-county area. Driving him or her crazy may end up driving you crazy for the entire time you reside there. Any interview is at the very least a good exercise in honing your people skills and building confidence.

Fast Fact

Interviewing mistakes on the employer's part:

• *Doing too much talking*

• *Making a hasty decision based on the first impression*

• *Giving too much weight to job-related negatives*

• *Spending too much time on irrelevant topics and neglecting job-related topics*

Even after you have successfully become employed, you should keep your resume up to date. Statistics show that we all will have at least four different job positions during our career. Keep your notes and job search data—you'll be surprised how useful it they will be in the future.

Interview Questions to Ask Your Potential Employer

Because this is a living document, please feel free to include other questions so you have something to keep referring to during your career, or to pass on if you develop a mentoring relationship.

Office Management Questions

- Who confirms the next day's appointments?
— *This may be something that the hygiene department is expected to do.*
★ *Usually the front office is in charge of all appointment confirming.*

- How long are appointments?
— *Anything less than 45 minutes is a red flag. You'll be tired and expected to do too much. Unless you're experienced and know how to stop if the presentation is something other than a prophy, you're in for some real headaches.*
★ *An office that allots 60 minutes for an appointment really values its employees.*

- Are uniforms provided?
— *Some offices ask that you change into your work clothes at the office. Some offices let you take the uniforms home for laundering.*
★ *Having the office launder the uniforms is the best of all worlds. Changing clothes really puts finality on your workday.*

- Are uniforms cleaned by the practice?
  — *OHSA requires that the office launder all outer garments. Some also launder scrubs worn under the jacket.*

- Is there a dress code?
  — *Some offices have everyone wear a specific color scrub outfit on a certain day of the week, so that everyone wears purple on Mondays, for instance. Some don't care what color you wear. Some pay for the scrubs, and some not only don't offer to pay, they expect you to wear business-type street wear under the lab jacket.*

- Who schedules the appointments?
  — *Most practices have someone to make appointments and answer the phone. If there is no one, or the doctor wants you to make your own appointments, the pay may be less. Valuable time is wasted because you won't be producing any billable procedures if you're making appointments.*

- Can you take vacation when you choose or only when the doctor is away?
  — *This can be a problem if you're a water skier and the doctor's a snow skier. Asking this question can eliminate of the possibility of time-off hassles later on.*
  ★ *In a one-doctor practice it's almost impossible to have this arrangement, but if you can get it, it's gold.*

- If the doctor is out sick or on vacation, are you allowed to work?
  — *In a large practice, this isn't usually a problem.*
  — *If the office is in a building with a number of other dental or medical offices, sometimes it's not a problem either. It's good to know the situation going in.*

- How often is the office closed for holidays, seminars, vacations, and other reasons?
  — *Large group practices don't usually close for anything other*

than a national holiday, but the smaller offices may close for a week during one of the big meetings like the ADA, Chicago Midwinter, the Yankee, the Holiday, or one of the many other dental conferences around the country.

★ *Getting paid for the week and having your expenses paid to go to the meeting is outstanding.*

- What holidays are you paid for, and must they fall on one of your usual working days?
  — *This is an important question. If your normal day off is Monday, and you only get holiday pay if the day falls on your normal workday, you won't be paid for some national holidays.*

  Some offices offer floating holidays where you can choose a different day off to make up for the holiday, they may just pay you for the day, or you may be flat out of luck and miss the holiday pay.

- What kind of recall/recare system does the office use?
  — *Recall systems vary greatly. There are no official names for any of them; they're as individual as the doctors or hygienists who invent them for their specific office. Usually, however, they involve some kind of postcard that is sent to patients, reminding them either to make an appointment or to keep an appointment that they made the last time they came in.*

- Does the doctor provide an annual review of performance and salary/pay?
  — *You'll want to know if you have to ask for a raise or performance review, or if everyone has a review at the same time, or if reviews are conducted on the anniversary of each employee's sign-on date.*

  ★ *An annual review on your anniversary date is the best. You'll never have a short year or a long year between reviews.*

- Is there a retirement plan?
  — *Also ask if there the employer provides matching funds. This is often figured in as part of your salary. So if you're offered $23 per hour plus matching funds at 3 percent of up to 6 percent of your salary, you'll know you can easily figure your contribution to the plan 23 x .06 = 1.68 per hour is your contribution to the plan. The company contribution, 23 x .03 = 69 cents per hour, .69 x 32 hours per week = 22.08 per week goes toward your retirement account from your employer.*

- How long until paid vacation is granted for one week, for two weeks, etc.?
  — *This varies greatly. If you get vacation time, it's not unusual to get a week after the first 90-day probationary period. This week can be used during the first year. During the second year another week is available, or some variation.*
  — *Those who work on commission usually receive an average of their annual commission pay for one week.*
  ★ *If you get paid based on production and also receive holiday pay, cross your fingers that you get this job.*

- Will you have an assistant to help you when placing sealants or doing periodontal charting?
  — *Usually you'll just have to pull someone in out of the hallway.*
  ★ *If the office has a dedicated dental hygiene assistant, you're in a good spot.*

- Is the dedicated assistant certified by the state?
  — *Some states certify dental assistants. If you live in a state that has certified dental assistants, it's part of your responsibility to make sure that person is licensed.*

- Will the doctor allow you to administer anesthetic?
  — *Even though it's legal in many states for hygienists to administer anesthetic, some doctors prefer to do it themselves. If the doctor encourages you to do all the injections in the*

office, make sure you don't have to beg someone to clean your room and seat your patients to make up the time. Don't get flattered that he or she is asking you. They may not be good at it and be relieved that there is someone else in the office who can do that nasty job.

★ *If you're encouraged to do many injections, your production and your value to the practice increase.*

- If you will be on commission, is there a base pay?
  — *If the office pays according to production, then it's likely that there will be an hourly base pay. The balance will be paid to you at the end of the month. This base pay is usually set low, so that you can easily go over that hourly base.*

- How much non-clinical time will be required?
  — *Will you be asked to do marketing?*
  — *Will the office be attending any meetings outside of your city?*
  — *Is the doctor affiliated with a nursing home, long-term care facility, or hospital where you'll have the opportunity to support him/her?*

- Do you have the flexibility in your schedule to lengthen or shorten recall/recare appointments as necessary?
  — *You'll find while practicing that you'll have some patients who won't need much of your time. Someone who has excellent oral hygiene and no restorations is one example, or a patient with clean dentures and six lower anterior teeth is another, they may need only 30 minutes. If you're working on hourly appointments, you will want to have some flexibility with appointment times. On the other hand, if you're working a 45-minute schedule and you have a patient that who loves to talk, it would be nice to extend the time to 60 minutes to give that patient the best care, and to make sure that they're comfortable and don't feel rushed.*
  ★ *Take all the time you need!*

- Is there a break room? Can you eat in or do you need to eat off the premises?

- Is there a cleaning service that cleans the office?
  — *Some practice owners expect the staff to clean up the office, vacuum, dust, and clean the toilet. Some have a service come in to do these tasks during off hours.*

- Is there a budget for hygiene supplies?
  — *You'll be surprised to find that some offices didn't even consider this. A budget for hygiene instruments and supplies is a must in order for you to provide optimal care for your patients. The follow-up question should be: How much is it? A $25 budget isn't exactly a budget at all when you consider that a single new hand instrument costs around $25.*
  ★ *Hand instruments should be replaced every twelve to eighteen months. They can be kept longer if the office has a sharpening machine for instruments.*

- Is there a budget for patient supplies?
  — *You'll want to know in advance whether you can give samples of floss, brushes, or other hygiene aids to every patient.*

- Are there any products or services that the doctor likes to promote, such as a certain whitening system, TMJ appliance, or cosmetic procedures?
  — *The doctor may have a special interest in orthodontics or one of a dozen or more things.*

- If you go on vacation, do you have to find a replacement hygienist?
  — *Unbelievable, but true. Some offices don't see anything wrong with asking the vacationing hygienist to find someone to take their place while they go on a vacation they earned.*

- If the statutes don't allow hygienists to provide direct patient care when the doctor is out, do you lose that day or can you come into the office to work on recalls, room maintenance, etc.?

— *While it's nice to have an unscheduled day off, monetary obligations often cannot tolerate it. Some offices will allow the hygienist to do office work, but may pay less per hour for the privilege.*

• Does the office pay travel time to continuing education courses, or just time at the course? (Make sure it's stated in the manual.)

— *Travel time should be compensated at the same hourly rate you receive for providing preventive oral care services.*

• If the schedule falls apart, will you be asked to leave for that portion of the day or possibly clock out?

— *You're an expensive employee to have around when you're not providing the services that you were hired for. Some doctors will fume just looking at you filing charts. Schedules do fall apart on occasion. For instance if it's snowing heavily, or raining with a hurricane bearing down, patients like to stay home. February and September are notoriously bad months.*

• How does the office handle emergency time off?

— *This might include days when you wake up in the morning too ill to go to work, or your child's school, or daycare center calls and asks you to pick up a sick or injured child.*

• What benefits are paid, i.e. uniforms, disability insurance, liability insurance, continuing education (CE), travel to, lodging and meals for CE?

— *Employment laws state that any required CE time, including travel, be paid time, and that other expenses associated with the meeting also be paid.*

• Will you have a key to the office?

— *You may have to wait out a probationary time before receiving it.*

- How early can you come in or how late can you stay to do charts?
  — *If you have a key to the office, it's great to be able to come in early to go over charts and set up the room.*
    ★ *Getting paid for going over the charts is important. It's part of your job; you can't just see patients on the fly.*

- If you do a presentation for a diabetes group, will you get paid if the presentation is on behalf of the dental office? (If this is done on behalf of the office, this would be an employment law compliance issue, and the office would have to pay)

- Find out specifically how much time the office takes off during the year.
  — *How much notice will you have to find temp work (not all areas of the country have established temp agencies).*

- How many hours are considered full time or part time?

- What happens to benefits if hours are short?
  — *This can be a problem if your schedule continuously falls apart. If you continually have two- or three-hour lunches over two weeks in September, one of the bad months, you can easily dip below the minimum number of hours required for full-time benefits. Usually you can have one short-pay period, but not more than two in a row.*

- Do part-time employees receive benefits?
  —*Some offices offer pro-rated benefits to part-time employees. That is to say that if you work 20 hours, part-time, you get half the vacation of a full-timer, and half-paid this or that.*

CE Questions

- Are you paid for time spent at CE even if you already have the maximum number of hours required?
  — *Unless the CE takes place on your day off, it should be paid at your hourly rate.*

    ★ *Getting paid even if it's your day off is a nice perk.*

- Who pays for CE?
  — *Some practices have a budgeted amount; it may be nice to know what that number is.*
    ★ *Having unlimited CE paid for is like having unlimited chocolate with no carbohydrate consequences.*

- Who decides which CE to attend?

- Are the CEs limited to only dental topics, or do they also include more general subject matter that could be of use to hygienists?
  — *Communication*
  — *Women's issues*
  — *Professionalism*
  — *Neutraceuticals*

Practice Management Questions

- What are the rules for treating family members?
  — *Can you work your child in during regular working hours, or do you have to see him during off-hours? Also find out what family members will have to pay. Some practices are very generous and some ask that you pay the lab fee.*

- What are the rules for dental treatment for staff?
  — *How will you get your own dental needs met? Can you have a real appointment, or will you get squeezed in when you and the doctor has an opening at the same time?*
    ★ *Having your own appointed time for dental work shows that the doctor values you and that you truly value his or her work as well.*

- How is the hygiene operatory set up?
  — *Make sure that it isn't set up for rear delivery. Rear delivery is considered toxic for the back, neck, and shoulders of a lone operator. It requires the solitary practitioner to twist and reach in unnatural ways, causing severe muscle stress and fatigue. If*

the treatment room is set up with this configuration, see if the patient chair can swivel to allow for a different arrangement.

- What about adult fluoride?
  — *Find out now how the doctor handles the fluoride issue. Some want all of their patients on fluoride at every hygiene visit. Some don't understand the benefits and will be very hesitant to allow their patients to be over-fluoridated.*
    - ★ *Allowing your discretion for fluoride treatments on children and adults shows value for your education.*

Doctor/Hygiene Relationship
- Is there a morning huddle that includes the hygiene department?
  — *Every practice consultant in the USA today encourages the use of morning huddles. These allow the entire staff to have input on the schedule and share what is happening to the patients that come and go throughout the day.*
    - ★ *Including the hygiene department in this discussion is a great way to feel like part of the team.*

- Is there a periodontal therapy protocol? (This may be called SRP or scaling and root planning.)
  — *Sadly, there are some practices that still don't have protocols for treating periodontal disease. Finding one of these offices in this decade is a red flag. The doctor or office manager may assure you that you can develop your own protocol and that the doctor has been waiting for someone to take the lead, but in all likelihood, the doctor has misplaced faith in the toothbrush and floss and provides untimely referrals.*
    - ★ *An office that has a periodontal protocol in place, where the doctor advises you to mold it to your liking, is something every hygienist is looking for.*

- Is there a caries protocol in the practice?
  — *This is a rather new concept. Remineralization therapies are only found in offices where the doctor is on the cutting edge of dentistry.*

★ *You're in an excellent place if the practice has a specific protocol for remineralization therapy. The hygiene department of any office can actively treat carious lesions and even turn them around if found early enough.*

• How many patients a day are you expected to see?

• What are the doctor's priorities or main interests?
  — *Is the doctor high on perio, or big on cosmetics, or does he or she love endodontics? It's good to know up front. If you're not a big believer in cosmetic cases and don't feel that you can approach patients about the appearance of their teeth or smile, you should find out the answer to this question at the first interview.*

• What are the production goals?
  — *A good production goal for the day (in the year 2004) is between 800 to 1500 dollars a day. California is higher and so is Alaska, as the fees are higher. Stay away from offices that have very low goals or none at all. It shows that the doctor has no idea what the hygiene department can do.*

• Do you have to recommend a certain amount of treatment per day?

• How are emergency patients handled?
  — *Seen right away?*
  — *Scheduled for the next possible opening?*
  — *Who triages the appointment?*
  — *Does the doctor speak with the patient?*
  — *Is there emergency time available in the schedule?*
  — *There really are some offices where emergency appointments are scorned. The receptionist may even get nasty with patients in pain on the phone.*
    ★ *A good dentist takes care of emergency patients immediately and treats those patients as if they were his/her best friends.*

- What is the office policy regarding parents in the operatory when their child is in the chair?
  — *There's nothing worse than having a parent in the operatory parroting everything you say. The second worse thing is having the parent in the reception room dying to get in. There is no good answer to this dilemma. Just knowing the overriding office policy is good.*

- What is the office's emergency plan, and is it practiced/gone over regularly?
  — *This is OSHA mandated. An emergency plan should be in place and discussed annually.*

- Are there regular office meetings?
  —*This is important. Open communication is critical to a smoothly running office.*

- What is the practice policy if a patient refuses x-rays?
  — *Ideally, the patient should be dismissed from the practice. They cannot turn down treatment that is deemed standard of care, even with a waiver. Some doctors will do an exam; some will just allow patients to make their own treatment decisions.*
  ★ *If the office protocol in this situation is to confer with the patient and come to some kind of agreement, and then schedule x-rays for the next appointment, you've found a good office.*

- Are you expected to know and understand insurance codes and billing?

- What is the office policy for working on pregnant patients?

Premedication Issues
- If a patient is required to take premedication but doesn't, how do you handle that patient?
  — *Reschedule the patient?*
  — *Give the patient antibiotics at the time of appointment?*

— *There's only one real answer to this challenge. The patient must take their medication one hour before treatment. You can either give it right away and wait an hour, or reschedule the patient for another time when the antibiotics can be on board for the required sixty minutes. These guidelines were set by the overriding authorities on these issues, the American Heart Association (AHA) and the American Academy of Orthopaedic Surgeons (AAOS), and therefore must be strictly followed in the interest of patient safety.*

Periodontal Therapy

- Is the office conservative (inactively watches pathology) or does it advocate aggressive prevention, conserving enamel (fixing any problems before they become acute or lesions become cavitated)?

  — *Either may be outside of your comfort area. A mismatch here can be problematic.*

  ★ *The right answer is that the doctor is conservative by conserving as much enamel as possible. It's likely that this doctor has a broad knowledge of what's going on in dentistry today and may even have a caries treatment protocol for remineralizing early lesions.*

- Does the doctor wear magnification loupes and a headlight?

  — *If the doctor doesn't, we wonder about his/her clinical abilities and how he or she values his or her own health. Proper vision and lighting are on the way to becoming the standard of care in dentistry. Without them, the practitioner will be risking postural injury and sub-clinical results of restorations.*

- What is the doctor's position on amalgam as a restorative material?

Swift Tip

If the doctor starts telling you how patients are overmedicated with antibiotics and the incidence of SBE is so low from dental procedures that it's almost unheard of, continue to be polite. When you leave the office, seriously consider whether you need this particular job.

— This is a hot question, and you're sure to get a number of interesting responses. There may not be any one right answer, scientifically, but at least you'll know where the doctor stands.

* Who does the new patient exams—the dentist or the hygienist?
  — The doctor should do the exams first. No treatment should be delivered by the hygienist before the patient has had an exam by the prescribing dentist. Some offices have the hygienists do the information gathering for the doctor: x-rays, perio charting, charting existing restoration, and a cursory soft tissue exam. Then the doctor can come in once the patient is prescreened, or prediagnosed, and the appointment time is streamlined.

* What is the protocol for patients who haven't been seen for over three years?
  — This is also nice to know. A patient who has not been seen in the practice in over three years should be viewed as a new patient and have a treatment plan mapped out before seeing the hygienist.

* What is the percentage of perio patients in the practice, or seen per day?
  — This number should be between 40 and 60 percent. Current statistics show that the majority of people have some degree of gum disease. If the majority of patients in the practice are not considered periodontally involved, there may be a lack of early diagnosis.

Getting Paid

* If a salary base with commission is offered to you, always ask if it's likely that the office will be increasing or decreasing this commission percent or your target production.
  — If they don't know, then have a contract signed between you and the office that stipulates that it cannot be changed (decreased percent or increase production) without the agreement of both parties.

- Are you paid if the weather becomes an issue, i.e., if there are large accumulations of snow or other unforeseen problems and you can't get to work? Also, if the office is closed due to adverse weather conditions, will you still receive your normal salary?
  — *Often there will be some warning of impending weather trickery. Some offices ask everyone to take a schedule home with them listing phone numbers of the patients scheduled, so that patients can be contacted should the office close.*

- If you will be working on commission, find out how often fees are increased. That may be the only way you can get a raise.
  — *This is often true for people who work on production. Other staff members may get annual salary increases, but those on commission may not.*
  — *Hourly, daily, weekly, biweekly, bimonthly, monthly—how often do you receive a paycheck?*
  — *It's nice to know when to expect a paycheck and how your time is accounted for.*
  ★ *A biweekly pay period is probably the best you'll do.*

A lot of the answers to these questions should come up during the interview process. You won't have to ask all of the questions, the interviewer will be impressed if you have prepared some intelligent questions to ask. Having read the list of questions will allow you to naturally ask questions during the conversation and make you look as if you've been practicing for years.

Swift Tip

Amy says: I learned one lesson the hard way. I asked one office I was interested in whether they offered paid vacations, and they informed me that since the hygienist was not producing during this time, they did not. I figured that I wouldn't be taking much time off. I didn't find out until I started working that the office closes for at least four weeks a year, and it actually turned out to be seven weeks. That's nearly two months without pay. In my area there is no temp agency, so it's not easy to find employment to make up this amount of time. I don't know about you, but I cannot afford almost two months without pay. I have bills and a family to support, just like everyone else.

2

Different Types of
Dental Offices

There are a number of different types of offices. The six major types are general (restorative), pediatric, periodontal, cosmetic, prosthodontic, and large group practices. Working in each has its pros and cons. Try to match your temperament with the type of office as well as the type of person your employer would be. A person who loves children may not be able to tolerate the conditions of some of the children who come to the pediatric office. Cleft palates, rampant decay, and neglected children often are often seen in the pediatric dental office.

Insurance

You wouldn't think that the type of insurance an office accepts would have much of an effect on your practice of dental hygiene. It does. It's a tricky thing, and we thought it was worthwhile to share a few key points with you. One is that patients, more often than not, will only pay for their insurance premiums thinking that that payment is their total contribution to their oral health. They have the impression that if their insurance doesn't cover the service, it isn't really necessary. If you suggest a procedure that isn't covered, they think you're just trying to scam them into paying more than they should. It's a tough problem.

Another important thing to know is that dentists/employers will sign on as providers for plans that don't pay them per treatment. It's more beneficial for the practice owner never to see patients who are members of a particular plan. It takes a strong stomach to work in a practice that really follows the money on those types of plans. Following the money can mean that some patients will be allowed to make appointments before they leave, and others won't. Or that some people will have to wait longer for treatment, than others. Let us take you down the road of insurance in the dental office.

Different plans work differently. There are thousands of plans, and sometimes there are different plans for people working at the same business. If you have a very large company in your town, there could be a plan for the workers on the floor or in the field, another for the support staff, one for the sales staff, and one for the management—or it may be divided up into even smaller increments. Your job is to ignore all of that, do the exam, formulate your treatment plan, and present the ideal plan to your patient regardless of what kind of coverage they have.

They may not accept your treatment plan, nevertheless, your professional ethics demand that you give them the best you have. If they decline, you must give them other options. That's the short answer, of course it's far more complicated than that.

The offices that accept managed care plans usually try to keep costs down by decreasing the amount of time allowed for procedures. It's one way to make up the cost disparity, because the practice only receives a small fraction of what it actually costs, or would cost, if the doctor or practice owner charged what they wanted. The practice may only get paid 40 percent of the customary fee for the procedure. Since the practice owner agreed to those terms, he or she cannot charge the patient the remaining percentage. Therefore, it behooves the practitioner to spend less time, use less expensive materials, and do more procedures in a day to make up the difference.

Another way to make up the money is to persuade patients to have procedures that are not covered by benefits, such as cosmetic treatments. This bait-and-switch tactic is at least unethical, at most illegal. If the patient could benefit from vital tooth bleaching or full-mouth reconstruction, that's one thing. If the office practice is to offer those services to everyone who enters into the treatment room, that's another.

While this type of plan looks like it's horrible for the office, patients love it even though they may travel great distances to find a participating office. They are blissfully ignorant of this dark side of their insurance plan. They only see that everything is covered 100 percent. If it's not covered, they must not need it. Patients don't realize that if there is only one dental care provider in a 150-mile radius that accepts their plan, it's probably because the plan is a bad deal for the dental practice. Owners look to make up in volume what they lose in money or keep patients waiting for treatment.

It can be difficult for these patients to get appointments, because often the schedule is blocked to only allow a certain number of people with this coverage type per day or week. This directly impacts your schedule as a hygienist because the person you want to see once a week for periodontal therapy won't be able to get an appointment unless there are cancellations. That is to say, if you can skillfully explain to your patient that they need periodontal therapy, even though their insurance won't cover it and they will have to pay.

In practical terms, the hygienist working in this environment will be tempted to work too hard. Time is short in the first place, and you'll be presented with extremely difficult cases to add stress to this situation. Often these people haven't had insurance of any kind for years. Too often, this means they haven't had preventive or restorative treatment for a long time and they'll expect you to clean them up in 40 minutes, which is of course impossible. The majority have bone loss, or rampant decay. It can be extremely rewarding to bring these people to health. You just have to be smart about it.

Hygienists are often tempted to give away free services to these patients. Trying to do four quadrants of periodontal therapy in 40 minutes, and then running behind schedule, is a recipe for disaster. Muscle injury is in the future, and autoimmune illness brought about by stress will take you down. Not to mention the attitude of the dentist when you're running behind schedule all the time.

If your patient cannot afford adequate treatment, a compromise must be struck. Giving away periodontal treatments is stealing from the practice, and providing periodontal therapy without the patient's permission is battery.

Working under these conditions is possible and can be just as rewarding as working anywhere else. The smart hygienist will work within the limitations of the plan. If a patient cannot afford periodontal therapy, a prophylaxis is all the patient receives. Over time a relationship will be built, and your patient may find a way to afford proper treatment. Educating your patient is the key here, not overextending yourself. Use what you learned and come at the problem from a different angle.

Items that are often covered under these capitation plans are preventive and diagnostic. Prophylaxis, fluoride for children, annual x-rays, or a periapical film for a toothache are some examples of the services covered by these plans. If you have an adult patient who could benefit from an office fluoride treatment, you may be turned down because it isn't a covered benefit. Offer it anyway if you think it's necessary, and recommend it because it's ethical to do so. Some patients will follow your recommendations even if they have to pay for the treatment themselves.

A fee-for service office is one that accepts the type of insurance that will reimburse the office for the majority of the cost of a procedure. If the patient is a member of a third-party payment plan, the patient is expected to let the insurance carrier know what was done and will be reimbursed directly. As a service to their patients/clients, some offices provide support staff to help with insurance billing.

Fast Fact

The dentist who negotiates to be contracted with the insurance company agrees to discount fees for all treatment and procedures. If a dentist's standard fee for a prophy is $74, he might contract for much less at $45 for the PPO subscribers. Even though the standard prophy fee is $74, the dentist has contracted with this insurance company to provide the coverage for $45 and the dentist cannot charge the patient any more than this amount. By agreeing to the contracted fees, the dentist hopes to receive an increased patient load in return.

The owner of the practice sets the fees at an amount usually decided upon by polite conversation at a dental meeting, based on statistics in a magazine or a formula constructed by a consultant.

Traditional plans often cover the costs of procedures with some kind of schedule. Usually, 100 percent of preventive services, such as prophylaxis and x-rays, are covered by the insured's premiums. There is a second tier of payment for restorative work that is usually covered at 80 percent or so, and a third tier of payment at 50 percent, which covers large restorative procedures such as crowns.

Working as a hygienist in a practice like this is often a little easier. The patients often have a higher dental IQ and are usually willing to have any treatment recommended by the dentist or the hygienist. Because the fees are higher, the production goals are higher. This is the type of office best suited for being paid on production.

Usual and Customary Reimbursement (UCR) is a term you'll have to understand as you learn the ins and outs of daily life in the dental practice. The insurance company will pay the percentage of whichever is less, their endpoint or the cost of the procedure.

The term Usual and Customary Reimbursement leaves patients feeling as if the dentist overcharged them or thinking that the dentist's fees are too high. This topic brings heated debate between the doctors and the third-party payers. Patients need to know that they are the ones contracting with the insurer in this context, unlike capitation plans, where the provider contracts with the insurance carrier. Dentists are not held to the UCR at all. They can set their fees at any level that

Speedy Story

Amy worked in an office where the capitation on hygiene averaged out to paying $9 for an individual adult prophy. No, it's not a typo— that's $9. If the hygienist's average hourly wage is $25-$35 an hour, you can see how an office is losing money in the hygiene department. A hygienist in this sort of office may be expected to do an accelerated hygiene schedule — seeing more patients to produce enough just to break even. This type of office may not be able to provide its hygienists with equipment to use like a fee-for-service office can. Accelerated or assisted hygiene, when done correctly, is a refreshing way to work. But when it is used to make up for hygiene department losses, the result is repetitive stress injuries, burnout/ fatigue, and questionable patient care.

feels comfortable. It's not necessary for the dental office to be close to the UCR, if they can find out what it is, it's less of a hassle.

Here's an example of how UCR works: A patient's insurance company will pay 80 percent of the cost of an amalgam filling. If the dentist fee is $125 and the insurance company's UCR fee is $150, the insurance company pays 80 percent of $125, not $150. The patient will be billed for the remaining amount, $25, by the dental office.

On the opposite end, if the UCR is less than the office fee, say $100, and your office fee is the same $125, the insurance company will pay 80 percent of the $100, not the $125. So, the patient has to pick up the 20 percent of the UCR, $20, and the remaining $25 over the amount allowed by the insurance company, for a total of $45. To set the UCR, some insurance companies might survey fees in the area by zip code, and set their UCR fee to the average. Most insurance companies will not disclose their UCR fees. If the practice fees are lower than the UCR, the third party doesn't want offices raising their fees to get paid more. The reality is that the UCR is almost always less than most offices' fees.

Capitation plans pay the contracted dentists much differently. They send a check every month regardless of services rendered or procedures done. If one patient or 1000 patients from that plan are seen in that office in one month, the payment is the same. If the office provides 10 procedures or 10,000 in one month, the check is the same. The office gets a certain dollar amount for each plan person signed up with that dentist's office. Whether the patient had an appointment, or not, or whether they had treatment in excess of that dollar amount or not, the office gets the same size check.

Where there is no third party involved, creative financing, such as bartering, is sometimes possible. The practice owner may provide orthodontic services in exchange for accounting services for example.

General Dentistry

General dentists are beginning to embrace the term "restorative dentist"—they see themselves as restoring health to their patients. Working in this type of practice can be extremely rewarding. Patients of all types and ages come and expect great things. As a hygienist in this practice, you can have a major impact on an entire family.

Educating parents about xylitol, soda pop consumption, and how their own oral health impacts their children's oral health is a lot of fun. You can educate elderly patients on their second go-round of caries susceptibility and show them how to decrease their new level of risk. Handicapped patients, cancer survivors, periodontally diseased, systemically diseased, all restorative cases, and more will be part of your day. You will never have a day identical to the day before.

One of the drawbacks to this type of office is the broad base of knowledge the dentist and hygienist must have. Because you'll be in charge of the entire body, you have to know a lot about everything. In a specialist office you'll have to know a lot about that specialty. For instance, you or the dentist should be aware of the little-known fact that high blood pressure is a symptom for sleep apnea. A patient who is known to have high blood pressure and complains of being tired or falls asleep in your chair would be a good candidate for a sleep appliance, or a referral to their M.D. for some kind of workup.

Often, the reason that a patient is in the practice is because they have insurance, not because they value their teeth. Or, they will be a client of the practice in name only, which is to say, they only come in when something hurts. Sometimes a patient will come to the practice after years of neglect. They have a dental plan now and intend to use it. Their teeth are often in such disrepair that you'll wonder why they weren't in pain. They might exhibit root tips, root fragments, or facial decay that encompasses the entire facial surface.

On the other hand, they may not have any decay and no bony support. Periodontally, they may be in horrible shape. Educating this type of person will be challenging. Knowing your limits of practice will also be challenging. Some general practice dentists insist that their hygienist take all patients, even if the hygienist is apprehensive about his or her skills.

Speedy Story

We'd like to take a moment here to point out that dental phobias are seldom true phobias. The child's fear is learned as a result of being manhandled or otherwise poorly treated by a dentist, hygienist, or support staff. This is your chance to create a healthy dental patient or a poor one. Often, the time of day or a personality clash between patient and clinician is to blame for the poor behavior of a pediatric patient. Don't try too hard. It's not important to finish a hygiene appointment. The child can win—it's not the end of the world. Charge a fee, dismiss the patient, and try again another day. Try a different hygienist. Words of wisdom from a pediatric dentist: "I'm happy to be the second pediatric dentist. Sometimes it can be easier... I can say, 'I'm not that other guy,' and sometimes that makes a world of difference."

That can work for hygienists, too. Don't look at a difficult child as a personal behavioral project. Look at that child as a personal growth challenge for you. Let it go. The goal is oral health for the little one, not getting him to learn from you how to overcome his phobias.

Pediatric Dentistry

If you have tons of energy and love little kids enough to see past the limitations of the parents, a practice that specializes in seeing children might be your cup of tea.

Children of all backgrounds visit the pediatric dental practice. Some are there because their parents value specialized care, some are referred by general dentists because the case is too involved, some are referred by pediatricians, and others are referred by restorative dentists because the child is too young or unmanageable.

A case that is too involved for a general dental practice may be one where the child has many teeth with decay. For a number of reasons, early childhood decay can ruin a child's dentition. The most difficult part of this presentation is the parent, most often the mother. Your educational efforts will be mainly for her. Without sounding like a know-it-all, you will need to educate the mother on how decay happens. Often, the mother will insist that she brushes the child's teeth, and already does all the things that you or the doctor have recommended. It's difficult not to blurt out the generic cause-and-effect, plaque-equals-decay, statement.

This kind of scenario can tax your

people skills as well as your education. Dentists and hygienists alike seem to forget that caries is multifactorial. The child's saliva may need to be tested for buffering capacity. Mothers really want what's best for their child, and often they think that only they have the information to make decisions. In a pediatric dental office you'll be required to wear two hats—one for dealing with children and one for dealing with the child's parents. It will be up to you to make this a positive adventure for both. Your most important job is to make sure they come back.

Periodontists

Gum disease is a major cause of tooth loss, and treating periodontal disease non-surgically is our territory.

The treatment of periodontal disease has undergone quite an evolution. In the 1950s it was all about calculus. The 1970s and 1980s were all about eliminating bacteria and toxins and achieving glass-smooth roots. Today it's about detoxifying pockets using ultrasonic energy and locally delivered antibiotics. It's about treating gum disease as an autoimmune disease and a modifiable risk factor for heart disease, stroke, chronic obstructive pulmonary disease, rheumatoid arthritis, birth complications, and who knows what all else. It's the periodontist who is the real physician of the mouth.

Because of its highly interactive nature, periodontal disease treatments are better delivered by clinicians with some experience. Like it or not, newly graduated hygienists have a lot to learn once free from their formal educators. A truly excellent periodontal therapist has a lot of experience with patient education and reading people. The periodontal therapist in a specialty office has excellent clinical skills that a new hygienist must master in another venue. This type of hygienist should be one who loves research and understands a holistic approach to oral disease. Beware of accepting a part-time job in a perio office, since continuity of care is crucial in long-term perio patient maintenance. An office filled with part-timers is not functioning to best serve its patient/referral base.

Hygienists who work in periodontal offices must keep abreast of new theory, illustrative thoughts, and medicine. Technologies change rapidly in periodontal disease treatment. A hygienist who works in a periodontal office will be responsible for a patient's overall health. Periodontists don't do much pocket elimination surgery any more. They are doing adjunctive surgeries, such as crown lengthening procedures or tissue grafting or what is referred to as cosmetic surgery.

Cosmetic Dentistry

Cosmetic, or esthetic, dentistry is not a recognized specialty within the American Dental Association, like periododontics or endodontics. However, there are a number of associations or groups of cosmetic dentists that have rigorous standards for entry or status. Cosmetic dentists are artists and a whole lot more.

A hygienist who works for a cosmetic dentist may be required to take care of some amazing dental materials. Special care must be taken when instrumentating around margins and using specialized polishing compounds on esthetic restorations. Patients who see cosmetic dentists will spend thousands of dollars on their cosmetic restorations and cosmetic procedures. It's up to the hygienist to see that those restorations are cared for properly and never damaged with harsh instrumentation, incompatible materials, or chemicals.

Another benefit of working in a cosmetic practice is the variety of non-dental tasks available. Patients in a cosmetic practice come there to have cosmetic work done, not because they have insurance through their employer or because they are in pain. This level of patient care can range from implants, veneers, and bleaching to orthodontic treatment. Patients may have their maintenance care done at their regular dental office. Therefore, cosmetic practices spend a lot of time and energy on marketing. Often, if the hygienist is interested, he or she can be a part of marketing and advertising.

Marketing a cosmetic practice may entail attending seminars, such as

Speedy Story

Shirley worked for a dentist who maintained that he became a dentist to work on teeth. If the patient didn't have teeth, he didn't want them in his practice.

women's expos or health fairs, writing articles for the newspaper, donating goods or services to worthy causes, or a host of other things. For the right hygienist, this can be more fun than he or she ever dreamed. These extra activities, which are often carried out during evenings or weekends, are usually paid for at the same rate of pay you're used to.

Prosthodontists

Prosthodontists replace missing teeth. They make dentures, removable partial dentures, fixed bridges, and implants. As with any specialist, a prosthodontist relies on referrals from the general or restorative dentist. All dentists are capable of making or replacing missing teeth in their patients; some, however, prefer not to. This is just one of many reasons a restorative dentist would refer someone to a prosthodontist.

A patient may exhibit complications that the generalist may not feel comfortable working with. Perhaps the patient had some disfiguring facial surgery, and the regular dentist finds working on him or her too much of a challenge. It may be that the patient is difficult or that the doctor doesn't like doing those kinds of replacements. A hygienist working in a prosthodontist's office or any other specialty practice will see the good and the bad of the dentists in the area. This can be a problem, as professionalism demands that opinions are kept under lock and key.

A hygienist who works for a prosthodontist will help patients maintain their prosthetics. Patients spend a great deal of money on these replacements, and if they are not cared for properly, there is danger of damage not only to the prosthesis, but to the tissue it rests on and the teeth supporting or surrounding it. As in cosmetic dentistry, a hygienist will unlikely build lasting relationships with patients, as they are often only seen for a short period of time.

Large Group Practice

If you need benefits, a large group practice is probably the best way to go. Large groups have a number of qualities that entice a new graduate. Firstly, there are other hygienists that a new grad can learn from. It's daunting enough for a new grad to enter the working world and see patients on their own. To be totally, wholly responsible is something else. A large group practice can take that burden and toss it out the window.

In a large group practice, the hygienist can usually count on paid holidays, vacation pay, 401K, and most importantly, people to help him or her learn. The hourly pay will reflect the fact that benefits are certain. The office will be open even if one dentist is on vacation. On the other hand, this type of practice rigidly follows the laws of the state, and because there are so many people, things move very slowly. This can mean daily frustration if the hygienist is one who is always striving to find a better way to do the job.

Large group offices often can buy materials at great discount. This is both good and bad. If a material isn't working for a particular practitioner, it's often difficult or impossible to purchase the material that does work. Often, one person—who may not even be a clinician—is the buyer for the group. This makes it difficult to make purchasing requests.

Large group practices often have a high turnover. For dentists and hygienists who thrive in an ever-changing environment, it's great. Some larger groups have committees where hygienists can have a voice or opinion in decisions. Belonging to committees can be very rewarding. However, if the practice is spread out across the state, it may be difficult or impossible to contribute if the meeting location is hours away by car.

This type of practice often has a number of contracts with third-party payers—the alphabet soup of PPO, HMO, and DMO. (Further explanation of the effects that insurance plans can have on dental hygiene is given at the beginning of this chapter.)

Working in a group practice environment is a great way to learn the craft of dental hygiene. It's not for everyone, the appointments are short often 30 to 40 minutes for an adult. With proper treatment planning, good care can be provided. For instance, periodontal disease is characterized by bleeding. If the patient is bleeding, then there is no reason to do a prophylaxis. Given a full hour, hygienists feel obligated to forge forward and "clean the patient's teeth" in a pool of blood, because that's what they're there for. In a thirty-minute appointment, treatment plans can be delivered, and the patient reappointed for proper level of care. There are hygienists who try to provide a prophylaxis on a case presentation like this in thirty minutes and they become disenchanted and burned out rapidly.

3

Treatment Planning

T reatment planning is the most fun part of a dental hygienist's job. Looking a patient over and determining treatment options to help them achieve optimal health is exhilarating. Finding a secondary choice is also a fun part of the job. Often, patients cannot afford to look like an "after" picture, and it's up to us to find a happy middle ground within the realm of dental hygiene treatment.

Firstly, hygienists are obligated to do as the doctor instructs them to do. In a single or double doctor practice, the lines are blurred and rules are loose, because the doctor is on the premises. This doesn't eliminate their authority or liability.

The type of treatment planning you do will vary depending upon the practice or dentist's philosophies and patient base. Our advice is to find a dentist who shares your values on patient treatment. Some dentists don't want to offend their patients with the grim reality of the health of their mouth, opting instead to have their hygienists provide cosmetic care only. Some are very aggressive in terms of periodontal therapy, recommending it for every new patient who has 4-5 mm pockets. Ask questions about hygiene treatment planning during the interviewing stage. You don't want to be employed at an office where you and the dentist are not of the same mind. This kind of situation only leads to stress, burnout, and loathing the career that you worked so hard to attain.

Fast Fact

Patients new to an office will have more treatment recommended for them than patients who have been with a practice for a long time. To put it another way, the same oral conditions in a patient of record may be watched, whereas a new patient will have the treatment scheduled.

Working for a dentist who is less aggressive with periodontal care than you are willing to be may force you, as a conscientious dental hygienist, to provide treatment for free. There is no such thing as a bloody prophy. If the bleeding is excessive, the patient should be treated for that bleeding, for a fee. Doing more is stealing from the doctor. Although the laws are different state by state, most agree that the doctor gets to make the diagnosis. If you end up working for a doctor who you think under-diagnoses periodontal disease, it's best to try to educate him or her with facts, journal articles, and visits from the periodontist you refer to. More involved procedures cost more money. A prophy fee is insufficient to cover the cost of treatment for anything more than a simple prophylaxis.

Recommend treatments that can benefit your patients and they'll learn to respect your position. Sealants are beneficial at any age, and fluoride varnish can make a huge difference to an elderly patient living dependently. Look at the recommended treatment already in the chart. If the treatment hasn't been completed, remind your patient to schedule the appointment. Vital tooth bleaching is something most patients would be interested in, however, they may be waiting for their oral health care professional to bring it up. Make recommendations you're comfortable with.

Look at your position as a pre-diagnostician; you're in the mouth a lot longer than the dentist is, for numerous reasons. Finding work for the dentist is helping the patient have a healthier or better-looking oral cavity.

Look for open margins on old restorations, and use the intra-oral camera to show the patient and the doctor. Faulty crown margins are another place to look. Sometimes an explorer can't find the opening, but a scaler can. In the early years, hygienists can have anxiety over telling patients that they had treatment needs. At some point they finally realized that their condition was not a reflection on them, the patient/client was just lucky it was found before it became a more expensive problem.

The new patient exam is the most important exam for the patient. They should be able to get to know the doctor and some of the staff. There is some controversy in our mind about the new patient exam. There are hundreds, maybe thousands of offices around the country where the dental hygienist sees the patient first, does the screening, takes radiographs, charts periodontal pockets, and cleans the patient up before the doctor ever gets a chance to see the patient. This just isn't right. If hygienists work on prescription, how is it possible for the doctor to prescribe a prophylaxis for the patient, retrospectively? It can't be done.

There are a number of reasons why so many practices are set up this way: On the one hand, it's much less expensive for the hygienist do the information gathering, prediagnose, and remove deposits that can obscure the dentist's vision. It's logical. However, the laws of most states don't allow for this scenario, and rightfully so. It is the dentist who is liable here. This is the most critical stage of the doctor-patient relationship. This is the dentist's patient, not the dental hygienist's. What does make sense is for the doctor to do the exam, formulate a treatment plan for the case to his or her best ability, and make a recommendation for the hygienist.

A different way to conduct a first patient visit, and one that makes more sense, is for the patient to be scheduled into the hygiene department, where the hygienist takes the records, does the prescreen, reviews the health history, and then calls the dentist in for the exam. This way, the records are ready; films, perio, existing restorations and caries are charted, providing information that could help alert the dentist to potential problems. This allows the law to be followed more closely, the patient receives care from two licensed professionals, and the office makes the best use of care providers' time for the best production. The same hour or thirty minutes in the doctor's schedule doesn't produce very much. A full-mouth x-ray as part of a new patient exam does help the hygiene production.

Following the Doctor's Orders

The laws in each state are specific. Dentists determine what hygienists do for their patients. Much like a pharmacist must have a prescription to fill, hygienists do too. Some dentists are very advanced and will allow you to do things you never thought you'd do. Others are so old fashioned that you'll be lucky to do a tiny fraction of what you learned through blood, sweat, and tears during your college experience.

The letter of the law is that you must work by prescription whether your state has general supervision, direct supervision, or independent practice. The doctor calls the shots unless she or he delegates that task to you. In most cases, the doctor is in the treatment room down the hall and some of the lines are fuzzy when determining who's prescribing. He or she can come into the room at a moment's notice, so you're not really practicing without the doctor.

In the ideal world, the doctor writes the prescription on the treatment plan, so the hygienist knows exactly what to do at the next appointment. In the real world, there is an understanding that you will do what's best for the person in the chair. If the doctor prescribes a prophy and you find pocketing beyond what a normal prophy would entail, some doctors will want you to present the new treatment plan and just inform them at the end of the day. This effectively allows the doctor to prescribe retrospectively. The drawbacks of this approach are the ramifications on the future of the dental hygiene practice acts. Allowing the dentist to prescribe retrospectively will allow him or her to continue to work with laws that don't reflect the reality of dental and dental hygiene treatment.

Other dentists will expect you to call them back into the treatment room to inform him or her of the new findings and await a new prescription. Every dentist will do things differently. To follow the letter of the law, hygienist should call the dentist back into the treatment room for a new prescription before continuing treatment.

The Laws of Your State

This is the short answer to the problem of following doctor's orders: Know your dentist, and communicate. Know the laws so you won't be taken advantage of. In some states, hygienists must work under direct supervision, which means that the dentist must check over all the patients before the hygienist can dismiss them. Since this setup is so clumsy and nonproductive, dentists often give the hygienist the authority to finish the case and dismiss the patient. By going along with this seemingly harmless activity, the hygienist thwarts all attempts at widening the scope of practice to allow the hygienists of the state to move toward a more realistic scope. Why change the law if everyone is comfortable with it the way it is?

Understanding the laws will help you avoid litigation and increase production. If you know what you are allowed to do, and do it, the practice will invariably increase its production. If you are allowed to delegate procedures such as blood pressure readings and polishing to dedicated dental hygiene assistants, you can practice what you are licensed to practice, making you a more valuable team member.

One thing that many dental hygienists too often neglect is taking breaks during the day. Just last week, even Amy worked through lunch. You must take breaks during the day. If you don't, your employer can be fined, even if you decline your break. This is serious. It is a law that every state has, and it comes from the labor laws that were enacted to help protect factory workers from working ungodly hours. Often, the dental hygiene schedule doesn't offer planned breaks. The theory is that you can finish early, or that if a patient doesn't show for an appointment, you could take a break. That works if you actually take a break. What usually happens is that you have instruments to sterilize, or a room to set up. Examine your state's break laws. Wisconsin mandates a break of 30 minutes in six hours for employees. If you own the practice, you can work until you drop if you're so inclined; as an employee you must follow the laws of your state regarding breaks, and the doctor and office manager must make sure you're following them or the practice can be fined.

Communication

Communication is one of the most important aspects of your job. Communicating with patients is just a tiny slice of whole pie. Communicating with the dentist and staff are diet-buster-sized slices. We asked several doctors how they would like to be approached with a number of different issues, including how they want to be notified when an issue with a patient in the chair comes up. We found that the doctors would like to be told before entering into the room for an exam. For example, if the hygienist encounters more bleeding or caries than usual or expected, a sticky note or a short conversation in the hall will let the doctor know that there is a surprise waiting for him or her in your treatment room.

Most scheduling or patient issues can be handled at the morning huddle. This is when the doctor, assistants, hygiene department, and front office staff come together for 15 minutes or so to go over the schedule and talk about the patients. A morning huddle is a good time to discuss bill payment, whether someone needs more or less time, if they have outstanding treatment unscheduled, or if there are other issues. Some offices have these meetings in the morning, and some have them in the evening just before going home.

The morning huddle is also a good time to review patients' insurance benefits. Offices that have routing slips printed up for each patient usually have some notation about the patient's remaining insurance benefits. Starting in September or October each year, it's helpful for the practice and for the patient to start looking at that number. If the patient has a crown on the treatment plan and has already met their deductible, it's a good idea to point that out during the huddle, so that it can be discussed with the patient during the treatment time. Having this discussion in the early autumn gives the patient enough time to schedule the appointment and have the treatment finished before the year is out. Depending on the procedure and the

Speedy Story

After years of changing recall intervals to suit the patient, Shirley worked in an office where she was called on the carpet for changing a recall from six to three months.

patient's deductible, this can be quite a savings for them. As a side note, it's profitable for the office as well.

Swift Tip

Start asking your patients if they would like to have their teeth polished. Most think the polishing step is critical to their well-being. They think that there's something beneficial in the polish; we are the ones who know better.

If you're having a problem with a staff member, the morning huddle is not the time to bring it up. If you're having some other kind of problem, this is not the time to bring it up either. Ask your employer for a meeting at the end of the day or over the lunch break so that you can have an uninterrupted span of time. Come with your facts straight, and come with possible solutions. Most dentists who have had any training in business or human relations will ask what you have done to remedy the problem. Don't say "nothing," or it'll be a short discussion.

The Dental Hygiene Treatment Plan

With all the talk about the dentist's treatment planning being equal to a prescription, you may be wondering what a dental hygiene treatment is. Really, the dentist only has to diagnose disease and mention a generic treatment plan. If the patient has a healthy mouth, the doctor may recommend a prophylaxis. If the patient has periodontal disease, the doctor may recommend periodontal therapy (often called scaling and root planing or SRP or quads). It may be up to the practicing dental hygienist to determine what to do during the prophylaxis or periodontal therapy appointment.

Prophylaxis

A prophylaxis appointment is probably the easiest work for a hygienist. A great patient-to-hygienist bond can occur during a prophy appointment. There is little need to discuss home care, there is little calculus to remove, and staining may or may not be present. A patient who requires a simple prophy may only need 30 minutes in your schedule. Your dental hygiene treatment plan would include PSR scoring, scaling, and cosmetic polish. If your patients do elect to have their teeth polished, use a mild or fine prophy paste. Look into the different prophy pastes. You may be able to save your employer money and save your patients' enamel.

Periodontal Therapy

The periodontal therapy treatment plan is a little more complex. There are a number of treatment issues to consider.

- Health history

- Pocket depths

- Amount of bleeding

- Host response

- Type of instruments available
  — *Sonic scaler*
  — *Ultrasonic scaler*
      Magnetostrictive
      Piezo
  — *Insert size*
  — *Hand instruments*

- Host modulation medications (Periostat)

- Site specific antibiotic therapy (See placement tips in Chapter 7)
  — *Arestin*
  — *Atridox*
  — *Perio Chip*

- Systemic antibiotic therapy

- Working relationship with a periodontist

Speaking in generalities is the most efficient way to address this topic, because there are so many variables.

Periodontal therapy is a definitive therapy. The concept of gross scale/fine scale is passé and has been for decades. If a diagnosis cannot be made, an appointment may be required to remove the gross deposits. This requires the use of a large ultrasonic insert or sonic scaler. Assistants are helpful with this level of debridement, to suction the large chunks of supragingival deposits. The appointment should not last for more than 30 minutes. Any longer and the clinician will feel

Swift Tip
For those seeking information on advanced periodontal cases, check out RDH, Dimensions of Dental Hygiene or Contemporary Oral Hygiene.

obligated to remove deposits apical to the gingival crest, and that is giving away free periodontal therapy. After this short appointment, the tissue will heal and the dentist can make a more accurate diagnosis.

There have been many speeches given and articles written on the best way to approach the topic of periodontal therapy. You can access *RDH* magazine online at www.rdhmag.com where you will find numerous articles on the proper way to achieve plaque and calculus removal subgingivally.

Pit and Fissure Sealants

Sealants are the second greatest innovation in preventing dental disease to come down the pike since the beginnings of the 20th century. Fluoride was the greatest.

Pit and fissure sealants can prevent decay in the most vulnerable areas of the most vulnerable teeth, the six- and twelve-year molars (a.k.a. first and second molars). Choosing the sealant material may be the hygienist's job. Some states allow dental assistants to place sealants.

Assessing which teeth to place sealants on has become more and more definitive. Years of study have determined that proper sealant placement over incipient decay will arrest decay and is safe for the teeth. Practically, there is no good way to determine the level of decay on the tooth with an explorer. Many dentists have been dismayed at the extensive decay found under what they thought to be a properly placed sealant. Research has illustrated the cause to be an improperly placed sealant, not the fact that a sealant was placed on a tooth with incipient decay.

Fast Fact

American Academy of Pediatric Dentistry position paper on sealants:

- *Bonded resin sealants, placed by appropriately trained dental personnel, are safe, effective and underused in preventing pit and fissure caries on at-risk surfaces. Effectiveness is increased with good technique and appropriate follow-up and resealing as necessary.*

- *Sealant benefit is increased by placement on surfaces judged to be at high risk or surfaces that already exhibit incipient carious lesions. Placing sealant over minimal enamel caries has been shown to be effective in inhibiting lesion progression. Appropriate follow-up care, as with all dental treatment, is recommended.*

- *Presently, the best evaluation of risk is done by an experienced clinician using indicators of tooth morphology, clinical diagnostics, past caries history, past fluoride history, and present oral hygiene.*

- *Caries risk, and therefore potential sealant benefit, may exist in any tooth with a pit or fissure, at any age, including primary teeth of children and permanent teeth of children and adults.*

- *Sealant placement methods should include careful cleaning of the pits and fissures without removal of any appreciable enamel. Some circumstances may indicate use of a minimal enameloplasty technique.*

- *A low-viscosity, hydrophilic material bonding layer as part of or under the actual sealant has been shown to enhance the long-term retention and effectiveness.*

- *Glass ionomer materials have been shown to be ineffective as pit and fissure sealants, but could be used as transitional sealants.*

- *The profession must be alert to new preventive methods effective against pit and fissure caries. These may include changes in dental materials or technology.*

Newer detection methods are a boon to treatment planning sealants. The use of the DIAGNOdent®, DIFOTI®, digital radiographs, and QLF™ (Quantative Light Fluorescence) make placing sealants safer, and the clinician can be assured of a good result. These technologies assure that sound enamel is under the sealant, increasing its effectiveness.

Newer sealants on the market include a glass ionomer surface protectant called Triage. This sealant acts as a fluoride battery, providing a never-ending supply of fluoride to the surrounding tooth. It flows nicely and bonds directly to the tooth, eliminating the need for etching. Triage is also hydrophilic, meaning you can place it in a wet field. The tooth shouldn't be in a puddle of saliva, but it doesn't have to be desiccated as it would for resin sealants.

Keeping up on new technologies is important, as we see with the changes in periodontal therapy and sealant placement.

Codes

The codes we use in dentistry are important to understand, and because they are so important as a whole they are very complicated. Some are simple and straightforward, such as code 330 for a panographic radiograph. Others are very complex because they don't reflect what we have done. The periodontal codes are the most non-descriptive for the generalist dental hygienist, because more often than not the patients have a presentation that spans health and disease. Decay on the buccal of tooth number 19 is clear-cut. A patient with periodontal disease around the lower left canine when the rest of the mouth is in perfect health presents a problem. Understand that every profession that receives payment from third parties has insurance codes to deal with. They are not the most important thing in the world, though, and shouldn't drive treatment recommendations. Patients without dental insurance do not need to have things coded, although it may be necessary for the office software.

You'll find that insurance company plans don't cover certain codes, for instance D1330, oral hygiene instruction. Use it anyway. the more often a code is used the more likely it will be a covered producure in the future.

D0120—Recall exam—Usually paid twice per year.

D0150—New patient exam—Usually paid out once for the initial exam. Can be used again if the patient was absent from the practice for three or more years.

D0180—Exam code available for use if more extensive exam is needed for a comprehensive periodontal evaluation. It can be used for new and existing patients.

D0350—Oral/facial images—Use this code when sending photos to

Fast Fact

When is a child not a child? When coding insurance for children, it's confusing to know when to switch over to the adult prophy code from the child prophy code. The going logic says that once a child has second molars, it's time to call him/her an adult. Children at this age still have childlike qualities, but their dentition is adultlike. For purposes of insurance coding, the person with fully erupted twelve-year molars is an adult.

the insurance companies for demonstrating treatment needs. This is most helpful with cases of very poor oral hygiene and cases needing gross debridement. If you have a camera, use it, and code it for the insurance company. This code can really help your production numbers. Patients will be more eager to accept treatment recommendations, and insurance companies may pay more often.

D0415—Bacteriologic studies for determination of pathologic agents.

D0425—Caries susceptibility tests.

D1110—Prophylaxis adult—Healthy periodontium. No bleeding, no appreciable calculus. This patient may or may not have decay or gingivitis. If you have a copy of the CDT-4 codebook, it will say that this code is for scaling and/or polishing. This description has been updated as of the spring of 2003, just two months after its publication, to read scaling and polishing.

D1310—Nutritional counseling for control of dental disease— Even if the practice where you work doesn't have a fee for this code, use it if you ever discuss nutrition with your patients.

D1320—Tobacco counseling for the control and prevention of oral disease—Don't use this code if you talk to your patients about the evils of tobacco. If your office has a tobacco cessation plan, use it at that time

D1330—Oral hygiene instruction—Use this code for every patient you spend time with on oral hygiene instruction. Some companies will pay on this code; others will not.

D1351—Sealant per tooth.

D2940—Temporary/sedative filling—Filling placed temporarily to maintain comfort for a short duration. This filling is remediable.

D2970—Temporary crown—In certain offices you may be asked to temporarily cement an interim or permanent crown.

D4342—Periodontal scaling and root planing—One to three teeth per quadrant. Often a patient will present with just a very few molars in need of periodontal therapy. This code, new for 2003, allows the practitioner to reflect what procedure was really provided at the appointment.

D4341—Periodontal scaling and root planing—This code is used to describe periodontal therapy of an entire quadrant. This code requires the office to also include which quadrant was addressed. If the clinician provides this therapy to a total of eight teeth in four quadrants, it is still often used, though incorrectly.

D4355—Full-mouth debridement—Enables comprehensive evaluation and diagnosis—This code can only be used if the debris is so gross that diagnostic evaluation can not be accomplished. A large ledge of supragingival calculus obscuring the view of the teeth fits this code. Large ledges of subgingival calculus do not exclude a diagnosis of periodontal disease.

D4381—Local delivery of chemotherapeutic agents via a controlled-released vehicle into diseased crevicular tissue per tooth, by report. The term "by report" means that someone in the office will have to provide a written explanation of why the treatment was provided. Sometimes it's the hygienist, and sometimes it's a member of the office staff who writes the narrative.

D4910—Periodontal maintenance. The patient has already had periodontal therapy and is being seen for the purpose of maintaining oral health. At one time, this code was expected to include the hygiene procedures and the dentist's exam. In 2003 it was revised to allow the exam to be charged out separately (code D0120).

D5986—Fluoride gel carrier—Used for a patient with rampant decay.

D7286—Cytology sample collection—Use this code for a brush biopsy. Some states allow dental hygienists to do this procedure; most don't. This doesn't mean that the hygienist cannot have the materials out and ready for the dentist to use.

D9215—Local anesthesia.

D9910—Office application of topical fluoride for root sensitivity—Can also be used for any other office-applied desensitizing agent.

D9911—This is for reporting adhesive resins, glass ionomers, or compomers for root sensitivity.

D9920—Behavior management, by report—Use this code for unruly children if a lot of time is wasted.

D9972—External bleaching—Per arch.

4

Networking

Once you are out in the world, the best way to network with other hygienists is to join the American Dental Hygienists' Association (ADHA). By joining the ADHA, you can meet other hygienists in your area through meetings, seminars, and CE courses. If you have some time to volunteer for your local component, you will help to further and protect the dental hygiene profession. Hygienists with whom you network can also assist you in finding an ideal position and learning which offices are desirable workplaces and which ones you should stay away from.

Professional organizations plan courses throughout the year, helping to facilitate completion of your CE credits for uninterrupted licensure. These organizations also provide structured networking and mentoring opportunities and offer opportunities for volunteering in your community to help those in need. By joining the ADHA, you will truly be a professional, whichever opportunity you pursue.

The sad fact is that across the country, only about 25 percent of all licensed hygienists belong to the ADHA. The biggest impact of low participation is the lack of bargaining power to maintain our legislative agenda. The ADHA needs members in order to protect and move the profession forward. The dental industry has a different perspective on patient care than hygiene has—it makes money on patients with disease. Hygienists get paid more if the patients have disease, but we get paid by the dentist. Doctors have a business to

Speedy Story

Kansas recently lost a battle to allow dental assistants to scale supragingivally.

run, unlike most dental hygienists, who focus on prevention and patient education. At times, the relationship between the two groups becomes adversarial due to the nature of the affiliation with disease, health, and money. As a professional organization, the American Dental Association (ADA) tries to protect the fiduciary interests of its membership, which sometimes clashes with the needs of dental hygiene. Nearly 80 percent of all dentists belong to the ADA, making their lobbying efforts much more impressive to legislative bodies.

You may not agree with everything that the ADHA does, you have no chance to help make progress by standing on the outside. When it all comes down to it, the ADHA is *our* professional organization. It is *our* collective voice. Think about this: If legislation that negatively affects registered dental hygienists is set to pass, legislators are not going to take the pronouncements of the hygiene population seriously. This happens every year in a number of states. If three-quarters of the hygienists didn't care, why should the legislators?

Even if you do not have time at this moment to volunteer your time to the ADHA, you can still join. Your monetary contribution will make it easier to attain legislative goals. Your membership does count! Raw numbers mean a lot when working towards legislative evolution. The more members, the bigger the impact the association has. The more members, the stronger the association is. You worked long and hard to attain your degree—protect it by belonging to an association that is engaged in developing our profession. You will protect your career, plain and simple. Not joining slows professional advancement. Without members, the ADHA does not have a strong voice or the finances to fight for legislation that will protect us all.

The ADHA has various payment options to help those who cannot afford to pay the annual dues in one payment. You can arrange to pay in quarterly installments. Please visit the ADHA Web site at www.adha.org to join.

Continuing Education Courses

You can empower yourself and your network even further by attending CE courses. Don't just think of it as a way to maintain your license. Think of it as a way to better yourself and meet people who share your interests. For each course that you attend, you are learning something new and gaining more knowledge, something that no one can take away from you. Even if you come away from a course with one new thing, you have increased your ability to grow and have improved patient care. By attending CE courses, you can get tips to practice more effectively and efficiently as well as network with hygienists who share your passion.

Take an ergonomics course early in your career. The term ergonomics refers to proper body mechanics to decrease strain, muscle fatigue, and muscle injury. In school, you are so focused on finishing requirements that some things, such as ergonomics, are neglected. Read ergonomic articles. You will learn how to practice safely and effectively from the beginning of your career. Sound ergonomic behaviors are the key to practicing without pain for as long as you want to. Neglecting ergonomics can cut your career short, with crippling hand surgeries, a torn rotator cuff, thoracic outlet syndrome, or fibromyalgia—not just carpal tunnel issues that so many focus on. The list is really endless.

Take a practice management course. Burned-out hygienists will bad-mouth these courses, but for a new grad, it will really help to learn the business side of dentistry. We all want to be the best health care providers we can be, and we all want to make a good salary. Sometimes we forget that it takes money to run a business. A dentist cannot afford to pay a hygienist a good salary unless the hygiene department is providing enough billable procedures to cover the overhead. A course can help you to learn how to code certain procedures that can optimize the treatment you are doing in your office.

Consider taking an instrumentation course. Refreshing your knowledge of instrumentation outside of the stressful environment of school might help to reinforce things you already knew. It might help you to feel more confident in your skills. You might learn some procedures or tricks that you weren't taught in school.

Attend one of the big conferences like *RDH* magazine's "Under One Roof," which is held across the country. This seminar is geared exclusively to registered dental hygienists. You will network with hygienists from across the continent. It truly is a positive environment! Other bonuses are that you can visit different parts of the country, take some time off, and deduct the cost of the trip for income tax purposes.

Role Modeling

Once you have graduated, you can learn from the other hygienists who work in your office or in your area. With experience, you learn things that work efficiently on your own in everyday practice. Experienced hygienists are usually happy to share with you. Ask hygienists whom you already know or whom you have met at a meeting if you can observe them in the office while you are searching for a practicing position. You are using them as role models.

Most experienced hygienists, or even any of your instructors who practice clinically, are more than happy to allow new hygienists to come and observe them. Over time, the relationship can turn into a mentoring one, which can grow to be extremely rewarding. Role modeling and mentoring are ways for our profession to stay strong. To stand together and help one another increases personal worth, sometimes called self-esteem or ego, and most importantly, patient care. If everyone waited for knowledge to come to them through experience, medicine would not have progressed past mustard poultices and leeches.

Being a role model is one of the most difficult and rewarding things that we do as people. You never know who's looking up to you. It may be the neighbor kid, your child's best friend, other hygienists, and even dentists. Be your best person all the time. Character is what you are when no one's looking; unless you live in a cave, you never know when someone's looking.

Role modeling is different from mentoring. Mentoring is an active relationship between two or more people. Being a role model is a passive activity. The model may not even know they are a model to someone else. People look at others around them in an effort to understand their world. This doesn't mean you should never relax; it does mean that if you never go to another CE, or don't stay interested in your profession, another hygienist may see your attitude as a license to slack off too.

Dress well when you leave the house. You never know with whom you'll run into at the store, at the dump, at the horse barn, at your son's soccer game, or at the nail salon. Think of how you react to people who are supposed to be one way and then you see them in a totally different way out in the world. Does it make you feel less confident if you find your financial advisor out at the grocery store, wearing cutoffs that are too short with a rip on the backside and a shirt that's full of paint?

When you go to CE courses and see other hygienists, you're likely looking at them and they are likely looking at you. Always present yourself well. Some people are comfortable being the least common denominator, and look for people who are the easiest to follow. You might be that person, and it will cost you and your profession a valuable reputation. Working hard at achieving recognition for the worthy service we provide in health care delivery can all be wiped away by hygienists who don't take their job seriously.

Role modeling doesn't just stop at what you wear. Be diligent in how you practice. Make sure you read about all aspects of dental hygiene. Make sure you take care of your physical and mental needs by exercising, resting, and light reading or movie watching. Just don't let those pursuits get in the way of keeping up with the necessary things of your profession. If you work in a pediatric office, you don't need to know everything there is about cosmetic dentistry, just everything there is about pediatric dental hygiene.

Choose your role models well. If you get a job where the last hygienist had excellent paperwork, and you find the patients well educated, you are in a good spot. If the hygienist you are replacing got by with good enough, use that experience as a poor role model and find a way not to fall into the same traps. Don't allow poor attitudes to prevail or seep into your outlook. Take active steps to find someone positive to look up to.

In the real world of dental hygiene, some offices are the scene of a minor turf war between new grads and seasoned hygienists. This war manifests itself in the new graduates acting as if they are in some way superior. They act as if they have the only handle on what's new in dental hygiene; they perceive themselves as the only ones privy to the new science, or new techniques. The seasoned hygienists, on the other hand, behave as if the new crop of hygienists is ignorant of the real world, and they spend unneeded energy beating them down, squashing their enthusiasm, and creating other embittered hygienists just like they are.

The reality is that the lines are not drawn where we think they are. The lines are really between enthusiastic hygienists and those who are there just to punch the clock—not between seasoned and unseasoned hygienists. It may be that the instructors at a particular college are not really teaching new and improved dental hygiene concepts to their students. Because the students are hearing these things for the first time from a supposedly credible source, they have a perfect reason, nay, need, to assume that they are getting the best current information. The instructors may be as burned out as the hygienist you'll work with some day who has been doing the same thing for fifteen years. Some instructors are too cautious in waiting for more proof, and neglect teaching new ideas to their students. Proof isn't a bad thing. Maybe some information shouldn't be on the test, which is not to say it shouldn't be taught.

There are hygienists who read and study their profession, treating it as a thirty-year program, not just a two- or four-year educational commitment. These hygienists are hard to find, but they are out there, and it would be terrific for you to network with them. One great place to find such dedicated colleagues is an online dental hygiene group. There are many on the Internet look for the one with the most posts per month, not just the biggest attendance list. The site www.yahoogroups.com lists a number of groups for dental hygienists, the biggest and most active being the RDH group monitored by Amy at www.amyrdh.com.

If you find yourself working with a seasoned hygienist who has a burned-out attitude towards patients or the dental hygiene profession, steer clear. It's unlikely that you can educate them, they don't want to be educated. These hygienists are often the favorites of patients, because these patients don't want to be educated either. You should remember that educating patients is your number-one job, even if they don't want to hear what you have to tell them. That is not to say that you need to educate all of them in a single appointment. In time, you'll begin to recognize what your patients/clients will respond best to, and that's what you should talk about.

Mentoring

Firstly, mentoring is different from presenting one's self as a good role model. It is different in one important way. In role modeling, the role model doesn't always know who's looking up to them. In mentoring, the relationship is obvious. One party is looking to the other for guidance and advice, and the other is teaching and introducing the protégé to influential people and peers. Each makes the other look good.

In a mentoring relationship, the mentor encourages the protégé to grow beyond his or her zone of comfort to become a better person and a better professional. Mentors have frequent contact with their protégé to monitor success and to deal with the inevitable setbacks.

Once you have graduated, mentoring those who are still in school is very fulfilling. You can become involved with your local association's mentoring program and offer support to someone in one of the classes behind you. There are many ways to mentor, not just helping with classes. You can give positive encouragement to a student; remember how much you needed it? Helping others towards graduation is a great way to give back. If you didn't have a mentor during your time in school, try to help someone out of the goodness of your heart. Expecting students to figure everything out on their own is counterproductive, the profession grows by people sharing and learning from one another.

Mentoring is also a good way to begin networking. Dentistry is still what's called a cottage industry. That is to say, dentists start their own practices, apart from their peers. It's tempting to practice the way you find comfortable, even outside of the law or practice acts. It's not like medicine, where doctors work in a clinic or hospital setting. There, ideas and methods can grow, and evidence-based practices have a broad knowledge base as well as a clinical base.

As a cottage industry, each dental practice is isolated. Dentists understand the limitations of working this way, and how their experiences must be matched against other dentists' experiences. They join their professional association to be in contact with their peers, and as a consequence, they have a large amount of political clout. Hygienists working in this kind of cottage-industry environment can also find themselves isolated professionally. This isolation is deadly to mind, body, and soul. Networking is an important part of dental hygiene. Whether in person or online, reaching out and connecting with other smart, educated dental hygienists will really keep the fires of passion going.

Publications

In dental hygiene, you are what you read. If you're only reading *Oprah* or *People* magazine, you may be up on popular culture, but your patients won't benefit from your knowledge of who's married to whom or what's the latest or greatest color to paint your walls. Reading a wide variety of publications helps make connections between a piece of information that you already have and a new piece.

Unless you're independently wealthy, it's impossible to subscribe to all the journals with articles you'd find necessary to have. The next best thing is the library. Even public libraries have electronic access to some professional journals. Make a quarterly visit to your local public library to use their access to the journals, and make an effort to visit a medical and/or dental library every few months as well. You'll soon find that you're ahead of the game when it comes to the cutting edge of progress. When others have a comment on something new or exciting, you'll have something to offer besides questions.

The best way to make the most of your library time is to make a list of journal articles before you go. Do this by visiting Entrez PubMed at http://www.ncbi.nlm.nih.gov/PubMed/. Type in the topics you're interested in, and then add them to the clipboard. Organize the clipboard by journal before printing it out. Now you have an efficient list to use once you get to the library of your choice.

Having publications delivered to your office or to your home is a great way to keep up what's new in your profession. The most popular are:

RDH magazine—free subscription at www.rdhmag.com

Contemporary Oral Hygiene—free subscription at www. dentallearning.com/COH/subscribe

Dimensions of Dental Hygiene—free subscription at www. dimensionsofdentalhygiene.com/

The Journal of Practical Hygiene—subscribe at: http://www. mmcpub.com/jph/

Joining the American Dental Hygienists' Association automatically gets you two publications, *Access* and *Journal of Dental Hygiene* come quarterly.

Read; read all the time. Our world is progressing rapidly, and to sit by passively and watch it go by is a sign of apathy. Even worse is to live with the mindset that you've learned it all in school and there's no need to further your education.

5

Purchasing Your
Own Equipment

Some offices don't understand hygiene practice. If one unknowledgeable staff person has a tight hold on the practice finances, they can come between you and excellent patient care. Having your own equipment will eliminate that power struggle and increase your worth to the practice. The manager and dentist will view you as someone who is particularly serious about your career. If that intimidates them, they won't call you in for a second interview, which will be your good luck.

Purchasing your own equipment is a topic about which many hygienists have a very strong opinion. Some feel that the doctor/employer should take on the burden of equipment ownership. They would never consider making a major purchase on their own to assure the best patient care. Their thought is that they work for the doctor, and he/she is responsible for supplying everything from patients to prophy paste. After all, the doctor is the one making all the money.

The alternative mindset applies to hygienists who assume their own burden of professionalism. They work for themselves in a way, treating patients and taking full responsibility for their care. These hygienists want to work with equipment that they know and understand—equipment that works well in their hands. Being tethered to equipment from 1968, or being in a position of having to

Fast Fact

When you decide to purchase your own equipment, talk to the local dental supply rep and let them know you will be making some purchases with your own money. If you have a good relationship, it is possible to work out a payment plan or discount. Sales reps can also hook you up with representatives from individual dental companies and perhaps even loan you trial equipment. This usually applies to chairs, ultrasonic scalers, and larger items. It never hurts to ask, and building relationships with sales reps in the community is a bonus.

beg for new or updated equipment is not on the program. Dental hygienists have a license to protect as well as a professional obligation to promote patient health and a personal obligation to themselves to work safely. Hygienists also have an obligation to their families not to be so fatigued at the end of the day that they are unable to function at home. In today's world, achieving these goals is impossible with equipment that is decades old. New technology may look like a gimmick at first; in the end, it often becomes standard of practice.

Why would anyone want to work with substandard equipment? If you like working at an office but the instruments are not up to your professional standards, or if you are in an office that does not have the ultimate equipment, think of purchasing your own as a way to protect yourself and your career.

That attitude is professionally empowering. In some cases, you can also deduct the cost of the equipment from your income at tax time. In a perfect world, we would all work for employers who would provide us with everything we need. Let's face it, if the world were perfect, there would be no crime, and it would only rain when people were sleeping! The fact is that utopia simply does not exist. It may not be that the dentist does not want to purchase the best equipment for you—he or she simply may not be able to afford it at the time.

Although you're paying off student loans and are in a position where income is more critical than outlay, one major purchase a year can be achieved. While you are still in school, you may be able to get some equipment at student discounts. Take advantage of those! Companies can be very generous with discounts, and waiting until you graduate and get a job may put off the purchase for far too long.

These items can be purchased as part of student loans, giving you another edge. Something like magnification loupes will certainly last you ten or more years, making the investment just pennies per day.

If you're already out of school, you may want to consider a loan, too. Discuss this with your financial advisor; there may be tax advantages for purchasing at certain levels. We seem to get advertisements for very low-interest credit cards at least once a week. It may be smart to accept one of these cards to make the purchase, divide the balance by 12 months or whatever the low-interest term is, and then quickly pay it off.

What to Get First

To protect your neck, shoulders, arms, and back, a pair of magnification loupes is essential. These will make your job easier every day. Forget the myth that you will need eye correction after wearing them for a while; it simply is not true. For one thing, magnification loupes force you to sit up straight and not slouch. They will assist you in seeing, even indirectly with a mirror. Once you start wearing a pair of loupes, you won't want to work without them.

The most important and most useful piece of equipment for patient care is the ultrasonic unit. There are several varieties to choose from. Buying the least expensive model could cost you more in the end. Networking can steer you in the right direction for the best equipment. The basic thought process is that you need to have reliable equipment, and the best way to insure that is to get your own.

Hand instruments are also a good investment. Sometimes, it seems as if dental hygienists are the only people within the dental office who understand that hand instruments wear out. Without the benefit of a mechanical sharpener, instruments can only last about one year, or eighteen months at the most. A mechanical sharpener can extend the life of an instrument another six to eight months.

An ergonomic chair would also be a smart purchase. This will help you sit comfortably and safely throughout the day. Look for a chair that is fully adjustable, one that you can customize to your own body size and shape. The back should move up and down, in and out. The seat should be big enough to hold your whole bottom including your thighs. It should also tilt forward and back. The arms should reposition independently, moving in and out, up and down, as well as tilt. You may need a few weeks to get the chair fully adjusted, and when you do, you'll be well on your way to a long career practicing as many days as you wish.

Another wonderful and useful piece of equipment that you may want to consider is a handpiece, either ergonomic swivel or cordless. Polishing is a procedure that hygienists provide for nearly every patient, and having a handpiece that fits your hand, isn't encumbered by a hose, and doesn't require a rheostat can be part of dental hygiene heaven. Cordless dental hygiene handpieces are quiet, and don't sound like a dental handpiece does. Patients have learned to fear that sound, and like it or not, most hygiene handpieces do sound remarkably like a high-speed dental drill.

If you work alone, as the only hygienist in the practice, it may be worthwhile for you to purchase an instrument sharpener. A quality sharpener can increase the life span of your instruments and increase your effectiveness as a clinician. Sharp instruments are one of the most important pieces in the healthy hygiene puzzle. An entrepreneurial dental hygienist could create an income with a sharpening machine on clinical days off by going to friends' offices to provide a much-needed service.

6

The Typical Day

There really isn't a typical day in a dental office. There are no two days alike in clinical practice. One day might be filled with all the patients you wish would fall off the face of the earth, while the next day might be full of patients you wish you could trade your family for. A cute little boy will come in and tell you all about the magnificent benefits his new shoes have on his running and jumping abilities. A young woman will come in and tell you about her prom, or a fairy princess will arrive in your treatment room on Halloween. Clinically, the variety is also endless. It's never the same, really. Anyone who thinks dental hygiene is boring or tedious isn't living up to his or her professional obligations.

Take an extra 15 minutes at the end of each day to review charts. Even if you are not paid for this time, this will help you stay on schedule the next day. Print out the schedule for the day and make notes for yourself on it. Review who needs x-rays and exams and mark this on your schedule. Have these x-rays ready to go before the patient sits down.

Review the medical histories of the patients to see who needs antibiotic prophylaxis for artificial joints or heart conditions. If the front office hasn't called, call and leave a friendly reminder to the patient to take their premedication an hour before the appointment time. This will save any need for reappointing or for struggling with the dilemma of a dentist telling you to just give the patient their premedication at the appointment time.

Tips:

- Come up with a routine that is easy for you to remember. Stick with that routine for every patient so that you do not forget anything.
- Keep an organized room so that you do not have to run around to different areas of the office.
- If you have extra trays, get them set up for the day so that in-between time goes by more quickly.

Speedy Story

A patient was in for a first-time visit with Amy, a periodontal therapy appointment. Upon questioning the patient, Amy found out that the person had had a stroke and was taking a medication she had not heard of before. Only because the patient mentioned that it was a blood thinner did she realize its potential impact on her treatment plan. No one had picked up on it, because it isn't a commonly used anticoagulant. Amy called the patient's M.D. and found out that indeed, the patient needed to come off of this medication three days prior to any dental procedures. Not doing so might have caused a serious problem. Always check with your patients and look up names of medications if you are not familiar with them!

Always date everything you write or put into a chart. There are few things as frustrating, or scary, as finding an undated Post-it note in a patient's chart referring to a phone call or something less critical. You'll find that out soon enough. Even if you think you'll remove the note after the patient's appointment, date it. If the patient in question cancels the appointment, the note can be worthwhile for the next practitioner. Without a date, there's no way to tell if the note is twenty-four hours old or ten years old.

Updating Health History

Look for anything suspicious on the health history form before your patient is due. Make sure it's totally filled out; for unexplained reasons, some patients only fill out every other column. If you have questions, call your patient ahead of time and ask them to clarify.

Once you're finished looking at the health history, look at the films.
- Are they of good quality?
- Is the patient due for new films?

- How old is the full mouth series of x-rays (FMX) or Panorex?
- Does the past history of the patient require a new periapical film?

It is best to have the patient physically update a medical history each time they come in. Even if your front office doesn't want to take the time to have the patient fill out a new form, keep a form for yourself to have your patients fill out and sign in your operatory. You can even come up with a form yourself on your own computer and make copies. If a patient forgets to mention a condition and has signed a form without providing that information, you will have a stronger court case if complications present. Ask important questions.

- Since your last visit, have you been hospitalized?
- If you need to take premedication, at what time did you take it today, and what medication and dose did you take?
- What medications have you taken within the last 48 hours, including over-the-counter medications? List aspirin as an example. You might find that a patient has increased bleeding since the last visit. The bleeding may be attributed to a medication they have taken within the last few days before their appointment time. Keep abreast of all the new medications.
- Avoid asking questions patients can simply answer with a "Yes" or "No." Instead of "Have you had any medical changes since your last dental visit?" say, "What has changed medically for you since our last appointment? I see you were being treated for hypertension by your physician and were taking the following prescriptions."
- Ask them to list any herbal supplements they are taking. Certain herbal supplements such as gingko biloba, St. John's Wort, and garlic can increase clotting time. These supplements and others

can increase the effects of anticoagulant therapy. Your patient may not even know it can be harmful. Direct them to their pharmacist, who can cross-reference all of their supplements and prescription drugs. You will be doing them a great service.

- Ask patients if they have had any heart problems. History of Phen-fen or Redux use warrants an echocardiogram. One should be recommended, and the patient should be premedicated prior to any dental treatment until it has been done.
- Since the patient's last visit with you, have they been diagnosed with any new medical conditions?
- Have they had any surgeries, including outpatient procedures?
- Have a line for them to sign and date the form. You can set it up so that there are a few of these updates on one page to keep in the patient's charts.

If there have been *any* changes that cause some concern, always call the patient's medical doctor. If a patient tells you they had a heart problem and were in the hospital, it is also best to check in with the M.D. Their physician may not want them to be seen in the dental office for six months, barring a dental emergency, or may now want the patient to premedicate; the same thing may apply for a stroke. Some physicians will not want their stroke patients in a dental office, but neglect to mention it, or the patient doesn't hear that part of the recommendation. It's a scary time for the patient, and the rules and recommendations are lengthy. Some bits and pieces of information are not assimilated right away.

Some patients on anticoagulant therapy may or may not need to be off their medication before any treatment. Some M.D.s will not want their patients off their

Premed or No Premed?

Pins anywhere in the body usually don't warrant premed.

Breast implants can go either way; ask the patient's surgeon for a recommendation.

Shunts in or near the heart can go either way as well.

Brittle or uncontrolled diabetics may also need to be premedicated with antibiotics.

medication at any time because the risk-benefit ratio favors staying on the medication. To reduce bacteremia for these patients it may be helpful to have them using a power brush, antibiotics, and enzyme suppression therapy (a medication like Periostat) before beginning any treatment. Use power scalers on a patient with this medical history, and don't forget to use a pre-procedural rinse to decrease the bacteria in the mouth.

Antibiotic Prophylaxis—Premed

Premedication issues can be one of the most stressful situations for a hygienist. You might start working for a dentist who tells you to give the patient the antibiotic at the time of the appointment if the patient has forgotten. This is not an acceptable delivery method as described by the American Heart Association (AHA) or the American Academy of Orthopaedic Surgeons (AAOS). Stand your ground for the current standard of care. Do not treat patients if their physician recommends a premedication regimen.

Speedy Story

Shirley took a blood pressure reading on a female patient who was in her middle thirties and of normal weight. The reading was breathtakingly low, scary really. She wondered how the patient could be upright. After a number of tries with no increase, she took the pressure on the other arm, and it was normal. Shirley instructed the patient to go directly to her physician's office to have the nurse check her blood pressure, which she did.

Six months later, Shirley listened to that patient tell her that she saved the patient's life. That woman had had a tumor the size of a softball on her thyroid, which would have gone undetected even longer if Shirley hadn't taken her blood pressure that day.

Remember the importance of requesting evidence-based research on important treatment decisions. Ignoring standard recommendations is not worth the risk. Your doctor may insist that he is the one with the liability, and you will be held harmless, an actual term in law. It would be perfectly reasonable to ask your dentist if his malpractice carrier knows he is telling you to provide a service that goes against the reigning authority on premedication issues. Until the AHA or the AAOS change their recommendations, who are we to disregard them?

There are a number of places to get information on the recommendations from the American Heart Association regarding premedication for patients with heart problems, including. http://www.americanheart.org/presenter.jhtml?identifier=11086. For your convenience, we have incorporated the most pertinent details here.

Patients with high risk for Subacute Bacterial Endocarditis (SBE)
— *Prosthetic heart valves*
— *Previous SBE*
— *Complex cyanotic heart disease*
— *Surgically constructed pulmonary shunts or conduits*

Patients with moderate risk for SBE
— *Complex cardiac malformations (other than those listed above)*
— *Acquired valvar dysfunction (such as that caused by rheumatic heart disease)*
— *Hypertropic cardiomyopathy*
— *Mitral valve prolapse with valvar regurgitation and or thickening leaflets*

Dental procedures where antibiotic premedication is recommended for patients with high to moderate risk for SBE
— *Tooth extractions*
— *Periodontal procedures including surgery, closed periodontal therapies, probing, and recall maintenance*
— *Endodontic instrumentation or surgery beyond the apex*
— *Intraligamentary local anesthetic injections*
— *Prophylactic tooth or implant cleaning when bleeding is anticipated*
— *Initial placement of orthodontic bands*
— *Placement of subgingival locally delivered antibiotics*

Regimen for prophylactic antibiotic dosing for dental procedures

General prophylaxis	Amoxicillin	Adults 2g (children 50mg/kg) taken orally 1 hour before procedure
Those unable to take medications orally	Ampicillin	Adults 2g (children 50mg/kg) IM or IV within 30 minutes before procedure
Allergy to penicillin family	Clindamycin	Adults 600mg (children 20mg/kg) orally 1 hour before procedure
	Cephalexin or Cefadroxil	Adults 2g (children 50mg/kg) orally 1 hour before procedure
	Azithromycine or Clarithomycin	Adults 500mg (children 15mg/kg) orally 1 hour before procedure
Allergy to penicillin family unable to take oral medications	Clindamycin	Adults 600mg (children 20mg/kg) within 30 minutes before proceedure
	Cefazolin	Adults 1g (children 25mg/kg) unable to take oral IM or IV within 30 minutes medications before procedure
Patients do not need further antibiotic coverage. Patients who are taking antibiotics for other conditions must still take these recommended medications and dosages over their current antibiotic.		

Medication FAX sheet

Clinic _____ Fax number _____ Date_____

Dear Dr _____

Our mutual patient _____, DOB_____, is scheduled for dental treatment. The plan includes prophy, periodontal therapy, other, which has a high potential for bacteremia. This patient's medical history includes

_____

medications include _____. Please advise us on this patient's need for premedication as outlined by the American Heart Association, American Academy of Orthopaedic Surgeons, or the need for suspending drug therapy for a time.

☐ Premed according to the AHA or AAOS guidelines
   o I will prescribe
   o You can prescribe
☐ Please suspend _____ for _____ days before any invasive treatment.

Signed_____

I release this information exchange between my physician and my dental team.

Patient Signature_____

Thank you for your time in the matter of patient wellness. Please return this document via return fax to 1 555 555 1234. If you'd like to discuss this case, feel free to call 1 555 555 0123

Sincerely,

Dr. D. Donut
Donut Shoppe Dental

Recommendations from the American Association of Orthopaedic Surgeons

High incidence

— *Dental extractions*
— *Periodontal procedures—surgery, placement of antibiotic fibers or strips, scaling and root planing, probing, recall maintenance*
— *Dental implant placement*
— *Endodontic instrumentation or surgery beyond the apex*
— *Initial placement of orthodontic bands (not brackets)*
— *Prophylactic cleaning of teeth or implants where bleeding is anticipated*
— *Local anesthetic injections*
  ★ *Intraligamentary*
  ★ *Intraosseous*

Low incidence

— *Local anesthetic injections other than those listed above*
— *Rubber dam placement*
— *Oral impressions*
— *Fluoride treatments*
— *Oral radiographs*
— *Postoperative suture removal*
— *Restorative dentistry*
— *Orthodontic adjustments*
— *Placement of removable appliances, prosthodontic or orthodontic*

Regimens

Patients allergic to penicillin	Celhalexin, cephradine, or amoxicillin	2g orally 1 hour before dental procedure
Patients not allergic to penicillin, unable to take oral medications	Cefazolin or ampicillin	Cefazolin 1g or ampicillin 2g IM or IV 1 hour before dental procedure
Patients allergic to penicillin	Clindamycin	600 mg orally 1 hour before dental procedure
Patients allergic to penicillin, unable to take oral medications	Clindamycin	600mg IV 1 hour before dental procedure
No dose after procedure necessary for any regimens.		

Further, the AAOS recommends that all patients with joint replacements take a course of antibiotics before any dental treatment for two years post surgery automatically. Antibiotic coverage is also recommended for patients with what they call comorbidity, such as previous infections in a prosthetic joint, malnourishment, hemophilia, HIV infection, insulin-dependent diabetes, or malignancy. The third category for premedication for joint replacement includes patients who are immunocompromised, including those with drug- or radiation-induced immunosuppression. The *Journal of the American Dental Association* put out a paper in July 2003 that highlights the need for joint replacement premedication. We found a copy at http://www.ada.org/prof/resources/pubs/jada/reports/report_prophy_statement.pdf.

Time Management

This might seem like a logical step towards making life easier for yourself, but a lot of hygienists don't have a good handle on how to manage their day. The biggest way to help yourself manage your time is to know what's ahead. Patients are people, and people are full of surprises. That means start by going through your charts well in advance of your day. Either look them over the night before or come in to the office 30 minutes early to look at them before patients arrive. This is especially important as a new employee.

What to look for:
— *Health history*
— *Last films*
— *Last hygiene notes*
— *Treatment not finished*

On the health history, look for positive answers and see if they were followed up:
— *Did someone already look up the medications?*
— *Was the patient on a list for a hard or soft tissue transplant?*
— *What is the HgA1c number if the patient is a diabetic?*
— *Was an ASA level established?*

If they were followed up, you work in an excellent office. Congratulations.

All of these questions can be answered ahead of time. Make notes on the schedule you use so you can refer to them before you call the patient to the treatment room. When your patient arrives, take them directly to the x-ray room first, take the films, then go to the treatment room if it's in a different location.

Knowing your limits is a key to staying on schedule. If you're presented with a Class IV prophy, you're not going to get that person finished. Tell them so before you get started. If they have an involved health history that's radically different from the last

American Society of Anesthesiologists (ASA) Physical Status Classification

I *Normal healthy individual*

II *Patient with mild to moderate systemic disease*

III *Patient with severe systemic disease that limits activity but is not incapacitating*

IV *Patient with severe systemic disease that limits activity and is a constant threat to life*

V *Moribund patient not expected to survive 24 hours with or without an operation*

VI *Clinically dead patient being maintained for harvesting of organs* one, then it may be safest for you to reschedule. That's true for new graduates as well as hygienists who have been in practice for decades. It may be intimidating for you to dismiss a patient and ask them to reschedule to allow you enough time to address their special needs. The doctor may not be happy with your decision. It's up to you to educate your employer. Sometimes it's just not safe to treat people, especially if you feel as though you're out of your league.

Find time to take the blood pressure. It's an important part of the exam. If you live up north in seventeen-layers-of-sweater country, you may have to compromise and get a blood pressure sphygmomanometer that reads the pressure in the wrist or finger. While only 50 percent of the population comes to dental appointments, some of those don't go to the doctor. This screening can be lifesaving, and it's really so simple.

Scripts for Presenting Treatment

You may be thinking that scripts are for actors. What is meant by scripting in dental hygiene is a way of relating information to a patient in a well thought-out manner, one where you don't feel like you're grasping for information and the patient doesn't think you're doing a sales job.

One of the most frustrating aspects of our daily job is to explain why a patient needs periodontal therapy, particularly if they have been a patient of record for some time. Patients who have presented for years with bleeding on probing and feel as if that is normal for them are also difficult cases. Many offices today have periodontal or soft tissue management protocols in place.

We have included some scripts that should be helpful for you. They have worked for us. The danger in scripting is the potential for complacency. Don't develop a script for yourself and figure you're done. A script should be constantly evolving as new science filters in. Originally, Shirley's scripts involved explaining the need for glass-smooth roots for her patients. Today, removing that much cementum is considered over treatment.

Here's a sample of a script. This patient has been in the practice for some time, and doesn't like much of anything you have to do for her.

Patty Patient: Are you going to do that gum-measuring thing?

Heidi Hygienist: Yes, we are, sorry. I'll be as gentle as possible. It's important to know if you're losing valuable bone.

Patty Patient: I know, but it hurts. That's what makes my gums bleed, you know.

Heidi Hygienist: I know you think so. Here, look in this mirror as I do the measurements. If you see bleeding, it's a sign of active infection, not the rough hygienist.

Patty Patient: Whatever...

Heidi Hygienist: Does that hurt?

Patty Patient: No, not yet.

Heidi Hygienist: But look, see, there's bleeding there. The measurement is six millimeters. A dime is about one millimeter thick, so this is the equivalent of a sixty-cent pocket. (Hold the probe so the patient can see what the measurements are.)

Patty Patient: It doesn't bleed when I brush it.

> **Swift Tip**
>
> *Some patients will even keep talking, just to keep the hygienist off track and thus avoid hearing what they need to hear. If this happens to you, just make a note of it in the chart, so you or the next hygienist will make sure to say something. Your main function as a team player in an office is to make sure that the patient wants to come back. A patient who is sick and tired of hearing about flossing will not return until he or she is in serious trouble or pain. Learn to read your patients. If you do, you'll soon see that badgering won't work. Some patients cannot floss, and some cannot do as you ask of them. Try again next time, or shorten their recall to take the pressure off them and you. That's how you stay enthusiastic and willing to learn.*

Heidi Hygienist: I know. That's because the infection is lower than the brush can reach. Look, six millimeters is nearly a quarter of an inch deep.

Patty Patient: Jeez, so, wait. Why is it bleeding? I brush and floss.

Heidi Hygienist: You have an infection below the line that the brush or floss can reach, and as a defense, the body is trying to get rid of the tooth, seeing it as the reason for the infection. Your body is manufacturing infection-fighting compounds that are not only working on the teeth, they are affecting the whole body. That's why researchers are finding that periodontal disease, which is what you have, contributes to heart attack, stroke, etc.

Patty Patient: What do we do about it?

Heidi Hygienist: In our office we have a protocol...

Nice, huh? The patient in this example is co-diagnosing her disease. If you can have a mirror installed onto the patient light, you are one lucky hygienist. Just flip it down and the patient can see exactly what you want them to see. Let them see the manifestation of the disease.

Here's another example of a script that Shirley has used on particularly difficult cases.

The health history update is done; the BP is taken and noted. The patient is reclined in the chair. This patient has been advised about bleeding and consequences of the disease nearly every single time she's been in. Last time, Heidi Hygienist didn't say one word. Today she will.

Patty Patient: My gums are still bleeding. I can't come more than twice a year—that's all my insurance will cover.

Heidi Hygienist: I'll see what I can do (smiling with her eyes).

Patty Patient: Oh, I can taste the blood.

Heidi Hygienist (raises the chair): I can't do this for you any more. (An inexperienced hygienist will de-gown and get the doctor at this point.) You have an infection in your mouth and it's getting worse. A bacterial infection. I'm here to help you maintain your teeth, and I cannot do it when I'm swimming in blood. It's dangerous for me and unhealthy for you.

Patty Patient: But, but... they always bleed.

Heidi Hygienist: And we've always tried to accommodate you. But you're losing the battle, and me cleaning your teeth this way is called supervised neglect. If you won't let Doctor Donut and me take care of you properly, we're going to refer you to a specialist. I'm in over my head here. (The inexperienced dental hygienist is listening to the dentist—or better yet one of the more experienced hygienists in the office use this script.)

Patty Patient: I don't want to go to the specialist. What's he going to do?

Heidi Hygienist: I don't know. All I know is that we're skating uphill, and losing ground. I don't want to be a party to your losing your teeth.

Patty Patient: Now you're saying that I'm going to lose my teeth. What other options do I have?

Heidi Hygienist: We can put you though our protocol for periodontal therapy. It's the same initial step the specialist will usually start with.

Patty Patient: Why should I go there then?

Heidi Hygienist: Well, in order for this to work you need to comply. Sometimes specialists have better compliance from the patients than general practitioners.

Patty Patient: What do you mean, compliance?

Heidi Hygienist: There are a total of six appointments, and they must be spaced out a week apart. You need to be committed to those appointments. We'll ask you to use special equipment, and possibly take medications.

Patty Patient: Equipment? What the heck!

Heidi Hygienist: Patty, we know what's best to keep your teeth in your head—that's where you want them to stay, right? Without a drastic change now, there's no telling how long you will be able to keep your teeth. You don't have many fillings, but your bone is disappearing. Without bone, the teeth have nothing to keep them in. It's not only about the teeth anymore. This level of chronic infection is detrimental to the whole body.

Patty Patient: But they don't hurt.

Heidi Hygienist: Gum disease is like high blood pressure. You don't know you have it until it gets really bad, or someone tells you. And we've been telling you for years.

Patty Patient: What if I still don't want to?

Heidi Hygienist: We'll refer you to another practice.

Hard words, tough stand. If the patient tells you to go ahead and just clean her teeth anyway, that she'll sign a waiver, don't fall for it. Those types of waivers won't hold up in court, a patient cannot sign away proper treatment. We are the professionals. They are the ones paying for our expertise and the judges know it, as do the defense attorneys. If anything unforeseen, or even foreseen happens, the patient's lawyer will probably win in a courtroom. We have to make sure that we take care of them in the best way possible, and we also have to protect ourselves.

That goes for premedication issues, too. Any patient who thinks they can sign a waiver to relieve you of your liability if they don't want to take their premedication, or wants to go against your recommendations, is wrong. We know the seriousness of not taking this precaution. If a cardiologist won't take his or her premed and wants to sign something, then go ahead, but that won't happen.

Here's an analogy that I heard recently that may help you converse with your patient about the different types of cleaning. This is not our original thought. The source has been lost.

Imagine you take your car to the car wash and the bottom rollers are turned off. The car gets washed from the bottom of the windows up. What more do you need? The hood and the windows are the most important right? You see the hood and need to see out of the windows. What do you care about the bottom half of the car? The part that accumulates the most mud, dirt, salt, and gravel, the part of the car that's the dirtiest, gets no cleaning at all. That's the same as only cleaning the visible portion of the teeth. The bottom part of the teeth, the part under the gums, is the place where the bacteria accumulate, where calculus grows. And that's the part you are willing to neglect.

Over time, you'll notice that you say the same thing to your patients as similar problems or questions arise. You'll have a script for manual versus power brushes; you'll have a script for office whitening; you'll have a script for why the other hygienists didn't say anything about a problem and you did. Most of these scripts come from within yourself, trying to convey what you think is most important about the question your patient asked you. We're going to provide a few more scripts here to cut to the heart of the matter of a couple of tricky subjects and questions you may encounter.

Where's the other girl (hygienist)?

Patti Patient: Where's the other girl? I really liked her.

Heidi Hygienist: She decided to get a job closer to home.

Patti Patient: Really? Oh, I guess she did have a long drive.

Heidi Hygienist: I'm not sure where she works now.

Patti Patient: I really liked the way she did x, y, and z. She was really gentle.

Heidi Hygienist: Many of her patients say that I'm just like her. I've been very happy to take her position. She treated her patients well.

Patti Patient: Oh, when did you start here?

Heidi Hygienist: About a week ago *(or whatever)*. She made excellent notes in the charts, and I feel very confident picking up where she left off in your treatment plan. *(Then add a little intimate detail from the patient's chart, such as a bad spot on the upper right, a good spot on the lower left, or make a comment on your patient's child's age. Something to let her know you've done your homework.)*

Patti Patient: Oh, she even wrote that down, huh?

Heidi Hygienist: She was very thorough.

Patti Patient: Well, you know better than I do.

Heidi Hygienist: I'll be happy to take care of you, too.

Why does one person get more cavities than another?

Patti Patient: I brush and floss and still seem to have a new cavity every time I come in here. My husband brushes only once a day, and he's done in under 30 seconds.

Heidi Hygienist: It's not fair, is it?

Patti Patient: No! How can that be? I work so hard on my teeth. It's just not fair.

Heidi Hygienist: The short answer is that his metabolism is different than yours. The bacteria in your mouth are more virulent than his, or he may drink more water than you do...

Patti Patient: He never drinks water!

Heidi Hygienist: Well, it could be that he has a different makeup to his saliva.

Patti Patient: We eat the same foods!

Heidi Hygienist: Right, if his body makes different saliva than yours, he's going to have less decay, even if he eats sugar all the time. It's a complex equilibrium. Any little thing can set off the balance to promote further decay or less decay. Let's see what we can do to shift the balance towards less decay for your teeth.

Why hasn't anyone ever told me this before?

Patti Patient: My gums have bled since I was a teenager.

Heidi Hygienist: Did anyone ever explain to you that this bleeding was a bacterial infection?

Patti Patient: No.

Heidi Hygienist: It is. The bleeding is a response to a bacterial infection of your gums. Without treatment, your body will start to eliminate the bone surrounding the teeth. Look at the x-rays. Can you see the bone loss?

Patti Patient: Why hasn't anyone ever told me that before?

Heidi Hygienist: I don't know. Maybe your last hygienist didn't have time to be up on the latest literature. I just attended another lecture that affirmed this theory. We have to get rid of the bacteria in order for your gums to heal. Are you taking any blood thinners or supplements on a regular basis? Are you ill with any diseases you didn't mention on your health history?

Patti Patient: No. What does that have to do with anything?

Heidi Hygienist: I just want to make sure the bleeding isn't because you're on chemotherapy or something like that.

Patti Patient: No. Why didn't anyone ever explain it to me before?

Heidi Hygienist: All I can do is tell you what I'm finding today with the knowledge I have today. We used to think that tooth loss was the only consequence of periodontal disease. Now, we know that treating chronic infections is increasingly important, since they have been shown to have a direct impact on heart disease, stroke, diabetes, and other systemic problems.

Patti Patient: I've been coming here for years.

Heidi Hygienist: Yes, since 1976. I'm sure the doctor appreciates your loyalty. The bleeding hasn't been noted every time for your appointments, however it has been noted. I think it's time, and I'm sure the doctor will agree, that we treat this disease aggressively now so that you don't lose more bone.

Patti Patient: What do we have to do?

Heidi Hygienist: The doctor and I have established a protocol for this level of disease. It is...

Should I get a power brush?

Patti Patient: What do you think about those new power brushes?

Heidi Hygienist: For you or for me?

Patti Patient: For me. I've looked at them in the store, and they seem like they should work.

Heidi Hygienist: They do work quite well. I think you would benefit from using a power brush. I'd recommend the Braun Oral B.

Patti Patient: I was looking at one that cost $100. What do you think about that one?

Heidi Hygienist: The Sonicare? That's the one I recommended for my mother. She has a lot of problems with her gums and her teeth. If you like that one, go ahead and get it. It's an excellent brush.

Patti Patient: Why is there such a broad price range?

Heidi Hygienist: Technology. The simple brushes are great for beginners.

Patti Patient: So I don't need the $100 one?

Heidi Hygienist: I don't think so. You're doing pretty well with the manual brush already. I think a power brush will just enhance your oral care a little.

Patti Patient: OK then. I'll get that Oral B brush.

Heidi Hygienist: I think you'll like it.

7

Tips and Tricks
of the Trade

This is the main reason you bought this book, isn't it? Learning how to use established tricks and short cuts to make the most of your time with a patient is a key component in decreasing your frustration levels at work. When it comes right down to it, tips and tricks come in a couple of different categories: scripts, time management, and knowing your limits.

Tips on Removing Calculus

- Try starting on the linguals of the lower anteriors, since this is a known spot for most buildup, and then proceed to the buccals of the maxillary molars.
- Use calculus-dissolving gel. Apply the gel, leave it for about a minute, and then scale away. On occasion you may need to reapply and rescale, but there are usually very good results the first time around.
- On patients who have a lot of calculus, anesthetize first. Remove as much calculus as possible with the ultrasonic scaler and a large diameter insert on high power: then apply the calculus-dissolving gel. It is very easy to use, directions are in the package.
- During scaling and root planing and/or curettage, sometimes a restorative instrument called a cleoid/discoid carver or file is effective for removing the remaining tenacious calculus.

Periodontal files are designed specifically for removing tenacious calculus by crushing and disrupting heavy deposits of it.

- Explore, detectable root roughness may not be calculus, simply the texture of the root. Sometimes it's best to let the tissue try to heal and document the possible areas where calculus could have been left. Evaluate that area at a recare appointment. Usually with healing and shrinkage of the tissue, the tenacious calculus can become visible and easily removed. Removal of calculus with minimum destruction or removal of the cementum is the goal of the skilled dental hygienist.

- Where ordinary ultrasonic inserts don't work using the Burnett Power-Tip, made by Parkell on high power works if the patient is anesthetized.

- Periodontists handle this situation by flapping down the gingiva and taking a bur to the calculus that could not be removed blindly with hand or power instruments. They gently shave away the darkened areas that were in question, removing only small bits at a time.

- Sharpening the instruments during the appointment or taking new ones may be of some help.

Tips on Treating Periodontal Disease

- In the late 1980s and early 1990s, we had available to us a very potent liquid topical anesthetic that gave nearly profound anesthesia. Sometime in the late 1990s the manufacturer stopped selling it. It can still be attained by contacting a compounding pharmacy and having it mixed on-site. Hygienists who used it during that time called it "liquid gold." The active ingredient is dyclonine. Each milliliter contains dyclonine hydrochloride 10 mg, chlorobutanol hydrous (chloral derivative) 3 mg (preservative), hydrochloric acid if necessary to adjust pH to 3.0-5.0, sodium chloride sufficient to render the solution isotonic, and water. Rinse with 5 ml of the dyclonine mixture for 30 seconds.

- You can apply a small amount of dyclonine on a cotton-tipped applicator to the soft tissue that is sensitive; as a rinse mixed with water or used in a syringe directly into the sulcus or pocket.

- Keep current FMX and charting handy.
- Use the ultrasonic scaler. Ultrasonic energy has been shown to increase healing and disrupt the biofilms below the gum line, and it is also less damaging to the root surface than hand instruments.
- The best hand instruments to use are Gracey 11/12, 13/14, 7/8, SH6/7.
- Perio Therapy Protocols
    — *Schedule 2—1¹/₂ hour appointments to debride and detoxify two quadrants at each appointment.*
    — *Schedule 4—1 hour appointments to address each quadrant alone (Code D4341).*
    — *Schedule 6—1 hour appointments to address one sextant at a time.*
    — *For scattered pockets, figure on one hour for every six teeth involved.*
    — *After anesthetizing your patient (Code D9215), remove large calculus deposits with the large-diameter ultrasonic insert on high power.*
    — *Once the big pieces are gone, switch to a slim-tipped right or left insert and debride the pockets, moving the tip quickly. Every so often, release the switch; then use the deactivated insert tip to explore the surface of the root.*
    — *Continue with the small insert until the root feels smooth.*
    — *Use the 11/12 explorer or the perio probe to look for calculus or roughness.*
    — *If roughness persists, continue with the ultrasonic scaler, or go to a sharp hand instrument.*
    — *Continue until the quadrant, arch, or area you intended to do is thoroughly debrided and no more debris is flushed from the pocket.*
    — *Apply locally delivered antiobiotics per manufacturer's directions (D4381).*

— *Bring the patient up, give home care instructions, and reinforce the process. They should already have another appointment if this is the first.*

— *At the second appointment, reevaluate the first section. If bleeding persists, apply locally delivered antibiotics to non-responding sites. Add a home care adjunct to encourage your patient to take an active role in his/her dental health.*

— *Repeat the above steps at each subsequent appointment.*

• Another way to approach periodontal therapy is called full-mouth debridement. You may have learned about it in school. The entire mouth is addressed in one single setting, or at least within a 24-hour period. All pockets are debrided, and the tonsils and dorsum of the tongue are disinfected with chlorhexidine. This appointment is usually three hours long. If done with a few brain cells designated to ergonomics and function, it can be a great way to treat periodontal disease without too much discomfort to the practitioner or patient. The steps to this appointment could be as follows:

— *Greet patient.*

— *Seat patient.*

— *Review health history.*

— *Evaluate patient's understanding of the treatment you'll be providing.*

— *Perform pre-op rinse.*

— *Recline patient.*

— *Evaluate oral hygiene (OH).*

— *Review OH (some people like to do this step with the patient upright).*

— *Deliver local anesthetic (D9215) to the first and second quadrants.*

— *Start with the ultrasonic scaler on the first quadrants.*

— *Move to the second quadrant.*

Fast Fact

Even the best clinician leaves nearly 50 percent calculus behind after diligent scaling using a combination of power and hand scaling. Our tactile sense is correct only 28 percent of the time!

> — *Anesthetize the remaining two quadrants.*
> — *Finish the second quadrant.*
> — *Move to the third and fourth quadrants.*
> — *Disinfect the pharynx.*
> — *Disinfect the tongue, and show patient how to use the tongue scraper.*
> — *Raise patient.*
> — *Review home care and aftercare instructions.*
> — *Dismiss patient.*

- Use anesthetic if the condition warrants it. Use the anesthetic that you and your doctor agree upon. Septocaine is hardly ever needed for this type of procedure. Some hygienists like to have all of their patients fully anesthetized because they are intimidated by a fear of causing the patient discomfort. Some use it because it gives the patient a sense that the procedure is different from a prophylaxis.

- A topical desensitizing agent, such as those listed under the Tips for Sensitive Teeth (pg. 110) section, can help if used before treatment. It may help enough that the patient will not need an injection.

- DentiPatch™ is a nice option in certain circumstances. It's a little patch of lidocaine that sticks onto the attached gingiva. Use denatured alcohol to prep the site so the patch sticks better.

- Refer to the periodontist if you feel overwhelmed by the case.

- Bleeding is not a good indicator of current disease. It's just the only one we have at the moment. If careful probing elicits bleeding and the patient is not on anticoagulant therapy, it's likely periodontal disease. DNA probes and other tests have been devised to give the clinician the sense of security needed to treat definitively.

- D4341 is the code for periodontal therapy.

- D4910 is the code for future maintenance appointments.

- Alternating codes D4910 and D1110 has been discussed ad nauseam, to no one's satisfaction. Technically, once a person has periodontal disease that involves bone loss, they are finished with D1110, because it is a preventive code and it's too late to prevent periodontal disease. Some consider alternating the codes to be insurance fraud, but this practice is pervasive and no one has been cited or arrested for this type of inventive insurance coding. Sometimes insurance companies will even downgrade a D4910 to a D1110. The problem is that there are not enough codes to address what we do and how we practice.

- Explaining periodontal disease to your patient is difficult. For best results, sit the patient up in the chair and use a script so that you are sure to get all the information in. Discuss x-rays and charting. Discuss health-related concerns, family history, blood glucose levels, and smoking habits. This can take the entire appointment. Some doctors will like this approach, while others will only see a wasted appointment.

- The ADA has excellent pamphlets for explaining periodontal disease. Contact them for a list at www.ada.org.

- Ibuprofen is a medication that not only cures a headache, it decreases swelling and inhibits prostaglandin synthesis, which decreases the pain response and prompts healing as well. Studies have shown that taking up to 800 mg of ibuprofen before a dental appointment can be very helpful for the healing process. Periodontal therapy can be more comfortable for your patient/client and easier for you.

- Use an end-tuft-brush to apply therapeutic mouthwashes.

- Bleach in the water jet device has been discussed by nearly every seminar speaker who deals with periodontal treatment. The proportions vary from a capful in a tank full of water to a more concentrated mixture. Dentists and hygienists around the country have been recommending this mixture for years. This is a good example of why we need to practice evidenced-based decision-making. In an earlier chapter we discussed how dentistry is still a cottage industry. Isolation makes dentists, usually people who enjoy scientific testing, try something out on their own to see how it works on patients. It may or may not work. Current research does not support using anything in the tank of the water jet device other than water.

- At times, you might feel root roughness with your explorer and instruments. Even the most experienced hygienist has areas that are confusing: Is it root structure or calculus? If you have gone over these areas many times with different instruments, it might be best to allow the tissue to heal. Chart the areas where you feel roughness to reevaluate at the next appointment. With tissue healing and less bleeding, it will be easier to remove a deposit if it remains.

- If a patient is hypersensitive and does not like using a sensitive toothpaste regularly, ask them to start using it two weeks before their appointment time. This may be enough to cut down on their hypersensitivity.

- If your patient doesn't respond to this level of periodontal therapy, an exam by an M.D. is in order. This patient may have a systemic disease that interferes with healing. Most often this is diabetes. Refer all perio patients for a diabetes test at the time of diagnosis. There are nearly as many people walking around who don't know they have diabetes as those who do know they have it.

- Refer to the periodontist if the patient isn't responding to your treatment.

- Refer difficult cases to the periodontist before attempting your periodontal therapy, and then refer back to the specialist once you're done with your portion of the treatment.

Swift Tip

Amy sees difficult perio-dontally involved patients on a daily basis. You can view her case studies at www.amyrdh.com. The Hu-Friedy black hub 100 for removing heavy calculus is a real blessing. She does not use this tip for regular prophy visits, but it works wonders on those heavy black ledges and heavy tobacco stains. To protect your hands and wrists when dealing with thick, heavy calculus, use your ultrasonic scaler to break up deposits before you do any hand scaling. Amy also has sets of the right and left insert, a beavertail insert, and thick and thin inserts.

Tips on Placing Locally Delivered Antibiotics

- For narrow pockets, use the mirror handle to squash the plastic tip of the Arestin® delivery system.
- Use Code D4381 for any of the products.
- Atridox® no longer needs to be refrigerated; roll between hands to warm.
- Only mix the Atridox for 30 plunger pushes, not 100.
- Do not overfill the pockets with Atridox or Arestin; they swell up a little with the crevicular fluid.
- Press the canula against the tooth to cut off the Atridox as you remove it from the pocket.
- Use a wet cotton-tipped applicator or 2x2 gauze square at the gingival crest to break off the Atridox as the cannula is removed from the pocket.
- Use the capillary tip from the Atridox package.
- New technology from Perio Chip® removes all barriers to placement.

Tips on Caries Protocols

- Remember that rampant caries indicate a bacterial infection and can be treated with chlorhexidine.
- Parents can apply chlorhexidine to small children's teeth with a cotton-tipped applicator.
- It is important for new mothers to chew xylitol during the first two years of their child's life to deter inoculating the child with caries pathogens.
- Caries Remineralization Protocol
    - *Use four to 12 grams of xylitol a day. That amounts to a minimum four servings of gum with xylitol listed as one of the first three ingredients per day. Xylitol gum is effective if chewed for five minutes. (For more information on xylitol see www.xylitolinfo.com)*
    - *Rinse with chlorhexidine twice a day for one week every three months.*
    - *Use gum with Recaldent™; as with xylitol, chew for five minutes.*

— *Use Lozi Flur*™ *fluoride lozenges. Low-dose, long-duration fluoride is critical for remineralization attempts.*

— *Apply glass ionomer cement to all carious lesions until teeth are ready for definitive treatment.*

— *Check saliva for buffering ability and pH.*

— *Patient should be on a three-month recall/recare with hygiene.*

— *X-rays may need to be taken more frequently.*

— *Check for saliva quantity and quality.*

— *Rinse with municipally fluoridated water numerous times a day.*

— *Apply glass ionomer surface protectant to all surfaces that are covered with biofilm (code D1351).*

Tips about Placing Sealants

- Use cotton rolls to isolate the lower teeth, one on the lingual, one on the buccal.

- Using a Dri Aid™ helps hold the cheek back and absorbs saliva to keep a dry field

- Use a cotton roll holder, sometimes called a garmer, to hold the cotton rolls in place.

- Make sure the patient's head is turned towards you. This allows gravity to pool saliva in one corner.

- Use high-speed evacuation, during the etchant rinsing, then place the bevel against the cotton roll to extract any moisture. This is more efficient than trying to remove a wet cotton roll to replace it with a dry one.

- Make sure the bracket tray contains everything you'll need.

- Make sure the curing light is very near, or touching the tooth being sealed.

- Glass ionomer surface protectant, such as Triage, can be used as a sealant in patients at very high risk of decay. (D1330)

- If using a glass ionomer surface protectant, wet your finger and press the material into the pits or fissure to increase retention and penetration.

- Use the DIAGNOdent before placing sealants to be assured that the tooth is sound.

Tips about Saliva

- Saliva quality is as important as quantity. For caries-prone patients, check salivary pH to determine the nature of the bacteria's environment.
- Patients with xerostomia from medications or disease can benefit from over-the-counter salivary substitutes or moisturizers, such as Oral Balance®.
- If xerostomia is a problem, advise patients to use SLS-free toothpastes. SLS is one of the foaming agents in most over-the-counter toothpastes.
- Saliva is important for remineralizing teeth; most salivary substitutes do not contain enamel-replacement components, so these should be replaced somehow. There are a number of toothpastes that contain enamel building blocks such as calcium and phosphates.
- If the saliva is acidic, find ways to alter the pH, for example by asking patients to brush with straight baking soda or Denclude.

Tips on Denture Care

- Place denture in a beaker of tartar and stain remover; then put it in the ultrasonic cleaner for 15 minutes or so. Rinse and polish using prophy paste or air slurry polisher to remove any leftover stains.
- Instruct patient to clean the denture with straight baking soda daily, using a stiff denture brush.
- Use pumice mixed with hydrogen peroxide.
- Use a polishing lathe with pumice and water.
- The ultrasonic scaler works well to remove heavy calculus deposits on a denture.
- Instruct the patient to soak the appliance or prosthesis in vinegar at home.

Tips on Removing Stuck Floss

- A little wooden wedge will open the contact to let the floss out.
- Try to loosen it with an explorer.
- A floss threader loaded with a double strand of floss under the stuck piece and lifted up, or snapped out of the embrasure works well.
- Pliers or forceps can work sometimes.
- In some cases it may be helpful to use topical anesthetic on the gum tissue before attempting removal.

Tips for Ergonomic Practice

- The best advice for a long term, carefree career is to pay attention to how you sit while working. Never twist to reach for instruments.
- Using instruments of varying diameter helps muscles relax during the day.
- Use a gauze square soaked in mouthwash to defog a mouth mirror for better vision.
- Use sharp instruments.
- Magnification loupes help posture. Make sure they are correctly positioned in every way. Poorly adjusted loupes are as bad as no loupes at all.
- Keeping instruments in individual cassettes increases their working life. When left in a pile at the bottom of an ultrasonic bath, they can rub against each other, which negatively affects the cutting edge.
- Having your elbows down at your side while you work will help eliminate shoulder fatigue.
- Do stretching exercises during the day for your shoulders and back.
- Use pre-procedural rinses before beginning to work in a patient's mouth.
- Contra angles are helpful to keep your wrist in a neutral position.
- Don't perch on the edge of the chair; sit all the way back.

- Chiropractors recommend that the hips be higher than the knees when seated.
- Time is an important factor for ergonomics; make sure you don't stress yourself with inadequate time allotted for procedures.
- Avoid scheduling difficult procedures back to back; give yourself a break in between.

Tips for Sensitive Teeth

- Therma-Trol from Schein comes in a little plastic vial. Snip off the tip, squirt it onto the gauze-dried tooth surface, and wait two minutes.
- Over-the-counter toothpastes work well for sensitivity.
- Make sure your patient isn't using a tartar control or whitening toothpaste, which can increase sensitivity.
- Dispense fluoride through the ultrasonic scaler during debridement.
- Proclude™ is an excellent product for desensitizing teeth chairside. It is a therapeutic polishing paste. Denclude is the home version and can be made available through the office. (D9910)
- There are a number of products that act as barriers which work well chairside.

Tips for Taking X-rays and Avoiding Gagging

- If you know your next patient is due for x-rays, have everything ready to go.
- Use double packs to save time duplicating films for referrals to specialists.
- Put a small amount of topical anesthetic on the edge of the x-ray film. At times, this is enough to stop the patient from gagging.
- Have the patient breathe deeply in and out of their nose while you are placing the film packet.
- Have the patient raise their feet while you are placing the film packet.
- If using the ultrasonic scaler and working without an assistant, ask the patient to hold the suction hose so that it does not constantly

hit the spot where it sets off their gagging. Patients don't mind helping out, especially if it means it will help them avoid gagging.

- Patients cannot sign a waiver to hold you harmless for not taking x-rays.
- Remain calm; the more agitated you are, the more your patient will gag.
- If you always cone cut in the same place time after time, automatically overcompensate by moving the head forward or back; you'll develop a new comfort zone soon enough.
- If you always overlap, automatically overcompensate when you're aiming the x-ray head and that should take care of the problem.
- Continual elongation or foreshortening can be eliminated by overcompensating on subsequent films. Add a little or take a little away on the vertical dimension for every film packet.
- Try pedo size or size 0 film packets for adults who have difficulty.
- Have your patient hum while the film packet is in their mouth. They can't gag and hum at the same time.
- Have your patient take a sip of very cold water prior to placing the x-ray film packet.
- Spray the patient's throat with Chloraseptic sore throat spray to numb it.
- A little topical lidocaine applied with a cotton-tipped applicator to the lateral border of the posterior third of the tongue also works well.
- A sprinkle of salt on the back of the tongue may also help.
- Educate your patient on how they are using their tongue. Most gaggers puff up their tongue and force it against whatever is new in their mouth. Hold the film in place and ask them to concentrate on not pushing against the film with their tongue. It may take thirty seconds, but once they realize how much control they have over their own gagging it eliminates a lot of fear of gagging for other appointments.
- Use photo paper to print out digital radiographs for referring patients.

Tips for Staying on Time

- Review the schedule and charts for the day
  — *Mark who needs films or exams on the schedule.*
- Preset the trays for the day.
- Follow the same routine for each appointment.
- Use scripts to relay important information to patients to reduce the chance of skipping something.
- Keep the room organized.
- Use Post-it notes in the chart to highlight important things; don't use a highlighter directly on the chart.
- Sample of a well-organized procedure:
  — *Meet and greet the patient.*
  — *Take x-rays and discuss problems.*
  — *Ask patient to update health history while you're developing the films.*
  — *Review health history.*
  — *Recline patient.*
  — *Finish applying personal protection equipment.*
  — *Perform oral cancer screening—first exterior, then interior.*
  — *Perform oral hard tissue exam:*
     ★ *Say the words "oral cancer screening."*
     ★ *Make notes as things come up.*
     ★ *Discuss oral hygiene.*
  — *Perio chart (at least once a year, try to alternate this with x-rays).*
  — *Remove hard and soft deposits with the ultrasonic scaler and hand instruments.*
  — *Polish if patient requests.*
  — *Floss.*
  — *Apply fluoride.*
  — *Call dentist in for exam.*
  — *Bring patient up to sitting position.*
  — *Review treatment needs.*
  — *Hand off to reception desk.*

— Remove chair cover inside out.
— Place all disposables into the chair bag.
— Carefully wrap the chair bag and put it in the garbage.
— Spray the countertops and chair with disinfectant.
— Bring the tray of dirty instruments into the sterilization area.
— Start the sterilization cycle for instruments and tray.
— Take the next tray.
— Wipe down the room, respray or use premoistened disinfectant towelettes.
— Set up the room.
— Greet your next patient.

Tips for Working with Children

- Be confident and friendly.
- To acclimate the child to the sounds and feelings of the prophy cup, polish their fingernails.
- Teeth can be polished while the child is on the parent's lap.
- For a very small, new patient the goal should be to get only one thing done, which could be having the child allow you touch his or her lips with your gloved hands.
- Give the child some options if need be. This could include allowing them to pick one thing to skip or one thing for you to remove, like safety glasses, gloves, or mask. If they're afraid of one of those items, it may make the rest of the appointment a breeze.
- Not every child likes fruit flavors; offer mint or toothpaste if they hate the polish.
- The major goal of the appointment is to make the experience a positive one so the child will return.
- If the child doesn't calm down within fifteen minutes, reschedule and ask that the other parent bring the child in next time. This can sometimes make a huge difference.
- Just because the child is crying, doesn't mean you cannot clean their teeth. It may be a response that they cannot control, but they may still be willing to try to cooperate.

- Let the doctor know that you're having problems. When he or she comes into the room, explain the situation, but put a positive spin on it by happily telling the doctor that Nathan let you wear gloves to look in his mouth today.
- Allow children to graduate to an adult-size toothbrush for having nice clean teeth.
- Ask the child to brush to the count of ten in each of the four quadrants.
- Children with braces may need to come in more than twice a year; don't be afraid to recommend it.

Tips for Relating to Patients

- Don't overwhelm the patient with too much information at one time. One or two new things are enough.
- Before educating the patient, remind yourself that you must motivate to educate.
- Understand the motivational level of the patient before you begin.
- Plan your approach.
- Review previous notes on patient education.
- Start by asking questions.
  — *Do ask:*
    ★ *What is it about flossing that keeps you from doing it?*
    ★ *Do you think you'd use a power brush?*
    ★ *How often do you use mouth-wash?*
  — *Don't ask:*
    ★ *Why don't you floss?*
    ★ *Why won't you use a power brush?*
- If the patient becomes defensive when you approach them about what you have found, apologize and find out what they

Speedy Story

Shirley had a couple of patients who were teenage girls, and saw them four times a year during the time they had braces on. Their mother would schedule their orthodontic appointment directly after their prophy appointment. Shirley would remove the alastics and wire, put the wire into an envelope, clean their teeth, and send them off. The orthodontist would put the wire back on later that day.

do want to know. You may have to wait until next time to broach the subject again.

- Show concern for conditions such as hard or soft tissue lesions.
- Speak softly—privacy is important. Show the patient respect by keeping their private matters private.
- Use inflection in your voice because the patient cannot see your face. Your voice quality and vocal variety are very important because communication is imparted by tone and facial expression. The mask obscures a large portion of that communication avenue.
- Use active listening skills. Respond to what the patient says to you without sarcasm—watch your tone.
- Walk patients out to the scheduling desk and explain the treatment plan to the scheduling person. This way, there won't be any miscommunication between the patient, the receptionist, and you.
- Collect articles on gum disease and caries from consumer sources. Sometimes these articles are more interesting for patients to read than something put out by a professional organization.
- Check out Dr. Mac Lee's book, *Nothin' Personal Doc, But I Hate Dentists* at www.ihatedentists.com. It's an excellent guide to explaining procedures, and you may also learn what to say in lay language.
- Suggest vital tooth bleaching before any work is done on the anterior teeth.
- Hand your business cards out to your patients. These cards should be supplied by your dental office. Use them for everything, including writing notes for your patients to take home.
- Hang your diploma on the wall in your treatment room. Most patients don't know how we got to be hygienists. They figure we graduated from high school and that's it.
- Have all procedures and protocols written up on office stationary. Give patients a copy as they leave. They'll have something to take home and read one more time. Some offices even have a

presentation on CD-ROM to give to their patients. You can add a number of photos, actual copies of paperwork they'll see, possible outcomes, a flow chart, costs, or any number of other things.

- Sometimes patients aren't truthful or don't remember the past correctly. If they come in with a story about how they've been seeing Dr. Cruller every six months for ten years and no one ever told them that they have gum disease, call that office. You'll often be surprised to learn the real story that's written in the treatment notes.

- Patients don't understand our dental lingo: caries, decay, and cavity all mean the same thing to us, but patients think they're all different. Explain terms if your patient seems confused.

- The same applies to periodontal disease: Some patients may think that gum disease is totally different from gingivitis and periodontal disease. This is your chance to educate them.

- Call your patients after a difficult appointment to see how they are doing. Most often you'll just leave a message on their answering machine.

- Studies tell us that patients like chitchat from their health care providers. Make sure to take time for some small talk with your patients.

Tips for Working on Ortho Patients

- Patients with braces do better with small brushes—either child-size brushes or end-tuft brushes.

- Use a rubber polishing point for brackets and large open embrasures. Prophy cups seem to break down easily on brackets.

- Brackets really shine nicely when you use an air slurry polisher.

- If the gingiva is inflamed, a toothbrush and toothpaste may be safer to use than any motorized method of polishing.

- For patients who have poor oral hygiene, and the orthodontist won't remove the brackets and bands, fluoride varnish helps decrease demineralization.

Tips for Working Latex-Free

- Discus Dental's ProActive Care prophy angles. The cups are 100 percent latex-free.
- Young Dental prophy cups come in a latex-free version.
- The glue on some prophy paste covers contains latex.
- Anesthetics with latex-free plungers:
  - *Articaine®*
  - *Septodont, Inc. (http://www.septocaine.com)*
- Check out the American Latex Allergy Association Web site (www.latexallergyresources.org), which includes lists of latex-free dental products and information on its A.L.E.R.T newsletter.

Tips on Polishing

- Use a soft, webbed prophy cup.
- Use a contra-angled prophy angle.
- Fine prophy paste does less damage to enamel and esthetic restorations.
- Start on the lingual of the mandibular tooth furthest from you. Do all the linguals with the patient's head turned toward you, then the facials. Rinse, and then do the maxillary teeth.
- KaVo has a new powder for use in an air slurry polisher that uses microsphere technology called Prophypearls. It's less damaging to the enamel.

Tips for Patients with Apthous Ulcers

- If your patient has chronic apthous ulcers, it may be due to the toothpaste they're using. Recommend Rembrandt® Canker Sore toothpaste, Squigle® toothpaste, or Biotene® toothpaste
- If removing irritating components of toothpaste doesn't help, ask your patient to have an exam by an M.D. This condition can sometimes be a result of Crohn's disease.
- Canker sores or apthous ulcers are not viral; they are located only on the unattached mucosa.

- Cold sores or herpes simplex is viral; it is never found on the unattached oral mucosa, such as the tongue or cheek.

Tips about Patients' Insurance

- Check the routing slip before the patient leaves to make sure he or she has used up all available benefits.
- Complete planned treatment before the end of the year to maximize insurance coverage.
- Flex plans allow the patient to set aside pretax dollars for some dental work; this must be used before the end of the year or the patient loses this money.
- Ask your patients who are close to retirement if they will be losing their insurance when they retire. If you ask two years or so before they retire, a full-mouth reconstruction can be finished before they lose their benefits.
- Cases that involve extended or particularly expensive treatment may benefit from an in-house credit system such as Care Credit. It allows the patient to pay off their debt to the company, and pay the dental fees when due.
- Insurance companies will not pay a claim that does not include all of the necessary documentation. You may be asked to write a narrative for certain patients.

In order to make the most of your experience in the dental hygiene workforce, align yourself with one company that has a number of products that you use. This will streamline ordering and help defray costs. The more you buy from one company, the better your chances of receiving a discount. Get to know the sales reps. They have an important job, and a long relationship with one person may get you the inside scoop.

Tips on Becoming a Prima Donna (or: How to get the rest of the staff to hate you)

- Only clean your own room if you're working alone.
- Never take instruments out of the ultrasonic cleaner; that's someone else's job.

- Always take personal phone calls during the day.
- Read *People* magazine cover to cover before allowing anyone else to read it.
- Cancel on CE classes just after the cutoff for refunds.
- Come in one minute before the start time of the office.
- Ask your husband to give you only diamond earrings as gifts so that you can wear them to the office—the bigger the better.
- Don't waste your education on putting new toilet paper or soap in the staff restroom.
- Go to the bathroom a lot during the day.
- Don't make coffee for the office.
- Brag to the office about your activities outside the office. Let them know you won first prize in bowling, your son is the smartest in the school, etc.
- Only spread gossip that you think will further your career. When others' gossip comes around, admonish the gossiper.
- When free samples come to the office, take them home before anyone gets a chance to see them.
- Never take your own radiographs or develop them.
- Never stay late.
- If you file charts, make sure that they're always in random order so everyone will stop asking you for help.
- If the other hygienist is running behind schedule, don't let that stop you from eating the cookies someone brought that morning.
- When emergency patients are stacking up for the doctor, make sure the assistants can't find you to ask for help. Sit in the manager's office with the door closed.
- Get a very fancy car to drive and talk about it every time the assistants look like they need help.
- Ask the reception staff to run printouts for you. When the printouts are ready, say you don't need them anymore.
- If you're running behind and the receptionist comes to see if you knew your next patient was there, give her a dirty look and berate her in front of your patient.

- Make all patients wait until you're finished with your phone call from your lover, and make sure they hear you.
- Never put the sterilized instruments away.
- Don't let anyone know you know how to run any equipment other than the hygiene handpiece.
- Call at the last minute to say you'll be late for work.
- Ask the receptionist to cancel patients every Friday afternoon so that you can have your nails done for the weekend.
- Wonder aloud how you will spend your big hygiene bonus: a new car or an island vacation.
- Talk about your college days incessantly, making a point to infer that only you and the doctor have degrees.

8

Feeling Confident

eeling confident comes with practice. There will be days when you'll feel like you don't have a clue what you're doing. Times when you look at an x-ray and see calculus that you left on a patient's teeth, or a patient will tell the doctor you hurt them, or they will complain that you told them they have gum disease, and all of this will ruin your day. It will pass. Over time, the good will outweigh the bad. Confidence will build, and if you work with a caring dentist-employer, you'll feel good about your level of patient care before you know it. In this section, we want to give you some final information about living and working as a dental hygienist.

Selling and Profit for the Dental Practice

The dental practice is a business. True, the business exists to help people attain, maintain, and strive for oral health. Those are the goals of the enterprise. But the fact is that any business also has to deal with essential economic issues such as rent on the building, your salary, and the salary of the receptionist and everyone else on the team. Supplies and equipment are also part of that harsh reality. The doctor and the hygienist are the only two people on the team who provide billable services to cover the overhead. The assistant and the receptionist can recommend a certain treatment or enhancements of treatment, however they cannot bill for services. For example, if the patient is scheduling for a restoration on an anterior tooth, a support staff person may suggest that the patient consider bleaching their teeth

Speedy Story

Shirley had a patient who kept looking at his watch during the appointment. She raced through, thinking the man was in a hurry and wanted to get going. She felt good about doing him a favor and getting done so quickly. It turned out that he was timing her to make sure she was doing a good job. Afterward, he complained to the office manager that she finished faster than any other hygienist and that he felt cheated! Since he was a lawyer and a patient of record, his opinion was taken seriously

before the definitive treatment so that the new restoration can match at a better shade.

We believe that while all this is true and important, a hygienist or a dentist should not recommend treatment based on fees. Practicing this way becomes unethical. The patient should decide what's best. A reality check on pricing, of course, is the cost of professional hair and nail care. People pay thousands of dollars a year for upkeep on their hair and nails without thinking twice. If they value their appearance more than their health, that's their problem. We can educate them, and recommend treatments that we think are the best for the given presentation. The rest is up to the patient.

The previous example is one reason it's difficult to make financial judgments for patients. Another is that if the price is set higher than the practitioner's comfort level, it's difficult to recommend the treatment, even though our perceptions of someone's monetary standing may be all wrong. Remember that Sam Walton, the founder of Wal-Mart, almost always wore farm work clothes, and he was the richest man in America for some time. He could definitely afford full mouth implants, *if* he needed them.

Thinking about the fee and production can limit some hygienists. Somewhere in their heads they're thinking that they are making money off other people's problems. That's true, but so is your gynecologist, and so is a plumber. Services cost money. It's best to just look at the person in your chair and say to yourself that they deserve the best possible care from you and your dentist; they deserve the best that money can buy. That's what you offer them, and they can decide whether they can afford it. If they balk, then a second or third choice for treatment must be offered, including the choice of doing nothing, and the consequences of each must be outlined.

For whatever reason, the word "selling" has some negative connotations. Consultants seem to talk about selling dentistry to patients/clients. Dentists often use the word selling when trying to encourage hygiene staff to offer more treatment. What they are really asking for is to have the hygiene staff recommend more necessary treatment. It is our job to recommend different treatments that are available. Patients don't know everything about dentistry—they can't. You do.

Think of yourself as the keeper of all the secrets of dentistry. You know what happens to an amalgam after ten years of service, and you know that you wouldn't want anyone you care about walking around with this or other harmful dental conditions in their mouth. You'll be amazed at the responses you'll get for recommending advanced treatments or even replacing barely serviceable restorations. Your patient may not know that the yellow crown on number eight with the three millimeters of recession and visible metal collar placed in 1982 can be replaced. Offer it this way: "Patti, what do you think of that front tooth with the crown on it?"

"I hate it. I wish I could get rid of it! I hit my mouth on the handlebars of my bike when I was ten, and I've had to live with this ugly thing ever since."

"You know, dental materials have really advanced quite a bit since then. Dr. Donut can make you a beautiful crown without any metal at all."

"Wow—but is it as strong?"

"It sure is. Let's see what he says when he comes in here to do the exam."

Speedy Story

Shirley had an octogenarian as a patient. She was a never-married nurse who worked for our soldiers in the wars. She was bright, articulate, and in need of a new lower partial; her upper denture was in good repair. They discussed the new partial, and she asked if she could change the color of the teeth, to which Shirley enthusiastically replied, "Sure!" Then she asked if she could lighten the remaining four lower anterior teeth. Shirley was surprised and tried to talk her out of it. Then she reconsidered and gave the patient a good deal on the cost of the tooth whitening. The patient was ecstatic with the results. Her teeth reflected her life and her mental age.

"Great! I just got new insurance that will cover a lot more than my old plan."

That's what dentists mean by selling dentistry, simply recommending treatments that the patient can benefit from. You don't know what their financial resources are, so you shouldn't worry one single brain cell about that. Your job is to offer the chance for everyone in your chair to have teeth that look like an "after" photograph in a textbook.

Sometimes, doctors are referring to hygiene services when they talk about selling in the hygiene room. This is usually related to periodontal therapy. Patients can benefit from Atridox or Arestin, direct-delivery antibiotic treatment for periodontal pockets. Sometimes it's hard to remember to make these recommendations; periodontal therapy is a difficult procedure, and providing that level of care is all-consuming. There is at least one pocket in your room every day that can benefit from local delivery antibiotic therapy. Setting a goal for yourself to recommend it once a day isn't really selling, it's stimulating yourself to offer the best treatment available to your patients. If no one presents with a case that warrants this type of treatment, then so be it. Overall, you'll be doing well for your patient and well for the office.

Over time, you'll start tying things together automatically. For instance, high blood pressure is a symptom of sleep apnea. Skillful questioning on your part will elicit information from an innocent check mark in the "yes" column next to this condition on the health history. Probing for information, you may find that not only does your patient have high blood pressure, he or she also is fighting fatigue, wakes with a dry mouth, and has a sleep partner who says they snore. This is the perfect opportunity to recommend a lab-made snore guard that your doctor is very interested in providing for patients. That's called a hygienist who is on the ball; consultants call it selling dentistry.

Dental Office Economics—Commission Wages v. Salary v. Hourly

Within each type of practice lie many similarities. There is at least one dentist in each, for starters. He or she went to a fine dental school and has responsibilities you're lucky not to have. The reason you have a job there is because the doctor has a practice. Your livelihood relies on that. Hygienists who don't provide services at a level high enough to compensate their own existence in a practice are either badgered or fired. Keeping an eye on your own production numbers is a fun activity. You don't have to have a contest with the other staff; it's just fun to see how different things can affect your production numbers.

When dentists have consultants come to the office to help it shape up or improve it, the consultants tell them that the hygiene department should be making $X per day and that the hygienists wages should be 30-35 percent of that daily production number. When tracking your own production numbers, you'll be amazed at the fluctuation. Once you get good at your job, you'll want a raise.

In order to maintain a viable practice, the doctor must make money. He or she has bills to pay: lab fees, equipment and instruments, and support staff wages are just a few of the things that are his or her financial responsibility. In a large group practice, a hygienist's production (as well as the doctor's) must generate enough revenue to cover the cost of support staff positions, including operations managers, office managers, controllers, bookkeepers, human resources people, and others.

In doing your job, consider all your legal duties, and perform them for your patients. In another chapter of this book, you can look at the list of dental hygiene codes available to use. Use them all often. Scour the practice acts and see how you can expand your dental hygiene duties within the law. Doing so will give your day more variety; most hygienists limit themselves to three of four regular duties. We're not advocating yearly full mouth x-rays. We are saying: Act as if excellent dentistry were free, and offer it to your patients. For the most part, it seems hygienists are altruistic and happy to give patients more than they're paying for. Maybe private practice is not the right place for that attitude. Hygienists like to earn money. They learn to rely on bringing home a paycheck. Dentists can't afford a hygienist who can't help row the boat.

Speedy Story

Shirley has a very good friend who worked at an office that didn't believe in having hygienists on commission. The doctor had always paid a straight hourly rate, and offered her friend the same deal: $23 per hour, 32 hours a week. This friend didn't want to work being paid hourly. She knew she could make much more than that on a commission basis. She persevered and convinced the dentist to try it her way for three months. At the end of three months, she took the following numbers to the dentist.

Commission v. salary	Old way $23/hr	New way $10/hr	Old way $23/hr	New Way $37.50
Hours/month	128	128	128	128
Production/ month average	$4000	$4000	$15,000	$15,000
Percent wage	74% (not 33%)	32%	20% (office wins)	32% (close to 33%)

Effectively, the old hygienist was stealing from the doctor. He or she is not fulfilling their end of an "at will" employment contract. If my friend only produced $4000, her wage would be $10 per hour if she agreed to work for the same 32 percent. If she worked for the same $23 per hour producing $15,000, her wage percentage would be only 20 percent. She knew she could make money for the company, and she didn't want to get the short end of the stick. The old hygienist was paid whether the patient/client showed up or not. If all she did was polish the patient's teeth and clocked in and out at the beginning and end of the day, she was making a good income, but her position would become unstable.

Asking for a Raise

Eventually, you will be in a situation where you'll be asking for a raise. Even if you know that you'll have a scheduled yearly review, you should be ready to prove your worth to your boss. In the beginning, you may have had a probationary period where you and the doctor came to an agreement on a salary, but once a year or under certain circumstances, you'll feel justified in asking for more money.

From day one, start learning to track your production. This task is one of the things that your instructors didn't really cover in your college classes, and it's very important in the real world. Your employer will know how many procedures you've done and how much money that has earned for the business. You should know it too, and if you keep track of it throughout the year, you'll be in a good position to make adjustments in your treatment plans or recommend more advanced treatments if necessary, so that you won't be caught short come review time.

Once a day, ask your office manager or the receptionist for your production numbers. He or she will be able to print them out with a couple of keystrokes on the computer. You can even ask them to show you how to print them out yourself, so you won't have to bother them. You can print out a daily, weekly, or monthly log. The weekly or monthly printout would be the most helpful to you. Watch for trends: Are you reaching your target goals? This isn't blind ambition—it's reality. Most patients need more than just a conversation and a polishing, what we call C&P services. If you're not reaching your goals, find out why. Ask yourself questions like these:

1. Am I seeing enough periodontal cases a day?
2. Could any of my perio cases benefit from locally delivered antibiotic therapy?
3. Could I recommend more power brushes?
4. Am I taking enough full-mouth series of films?
5. Are all my patients up to date on panorex films?
6. Do all of my patients have sealants?

7. Have I talked about TMJ therapy recently?
8. Have I asked my patients if they like the color of their teeth?
9. Are enough patients on a shorter recall/recare schedule?

You can also ask to have your production numbers arranged by procedure on the printout, such as the periodontal codes, sealant codes, whitening codes, and the rest. You can maintain a computer database, or just put your sheets into a three-ring binder. Do the math monthly; track increases and decreases by percent. That will help you compile the data for the conversation with your employer when it's time for a review.

Questions to ask yourself:

• *Are you on time for work?*

• *Are you adhering to your work schedule?*

• *Do you work well with others and help out if needed?*

• *Do you have expanded functions?*

• *Are you constantly striving to broaden your scope of knowledge and translate that knowledge into patient care?*

• *Are you a flexible individual —do you handle crises well, including changes in scheduling at the last minute?*

• *Are you healthy?*

• *Do you take your patients to another level of care?*

• *Do you test your doctor's willingness to progress?*

Those are the kinds of questions business owners want to know the answers to. They don't want to hear that you've been there every day, and came to the office even when you had a cold. That's nice, but it doesn't pay the overhead. Along with your personal production, your employer would be interested to know how much of the treatment you recommended for your patients actually resulted in appointments and follow through. If you talked about vital tooth bleaching to three patients a day, and none of them made appointments, that doesn't bode very well. If you spent a great deal of time explaining necessary treatment to your patients, and they didn't schedule, that says something too.

Maybe you can show a case acceptance increase over the last year, or how you were able to find a special deal on equipment online at eBay. Maybe the fact that you are a member of the American Dental Hygienists' Association saved him or her money on all the continuing education classes you took. Or the savings may have come because you have disability insurance through ADHA. You may also want to keep track of your out-of-office activities that affect the office. Did you participate in "Run for the Cure" and wear a tee shirt emblazoned with your doctor's name on it? Did you go to the nursing home, talk to nursing assistants about denture care, and explain what your doctor can do for the residents? How about online activities? Does everyone in the Yahoo RDH group online know what a great dentist your employer is? All that counts, so keep track of it during the year. It will help you prove your value to the practice.

Know why you deserve a raise on the level of a business owner, not an employee whiner.

Your conversation might go like this:

Doctor Donut: I think I'm going to give everyone the same raise this year, 2 percent an hour for everyone!

Heidi Hygienist: Doctor, I was thinking more along the lines of 15 percent.

Doctor Donut: I don't know, Heidi. What makes you think you should get more than the cost of living index? I pay for a portion of your health insurance, and I have the 401K match, plus I have to pay your social security.

Heidi Hygienist: Doctor, I think I can prove that I've increased production in the hygiene department by more than 15 percent since this same time last year.

Doctor Donut: Half of that was the fee increase—did you figure that in?

Heidi Hygienist: That is on top of the fee increase that we instituted last January. The fees for hygiene-related procedures went up an average of 8 percent, and the actual hygiene production went up 25.8 percent.

Doctor Donut: Well...

Heidi Hygienist: Doctor, I'd like to show you that I also initiated dozens of conversations in the hygiene room that culminated in elective treatment provided by you and by me. See here? This averages out to nearly one elective patient per day.

Doctor Donut: Whoa, I had no idea it was so high.

Heidi Hygienist: It was hard keeping track, but I did, and these results were surprising to me, too. After a while it got to be kind of fun, like a little personal contest.

Doctor Donut: Well, Heidi, this is impressive. I've always wanted this kind of reporting from my hygienists, but you're the first one in over a decade who has provided me with the proof I needed to give a real raise. Let me look this information over, and I'll get back to you on the raise.

Heidi Hygienist: Can I expect an answer by the end of the week? Maybe we could schedule a time on Friday when we could talk. I have some ideas about increasing some of these numbers even faster.

Doctor Donut: Well, we still have time today. What can we do to increase the production, in your estimation?

Heidi Hygienist: Well, I've noticed that we aren't always on the same page with our perio program, and I was hoping that we could come to some agreement to get better compliance from our patients to actually schedule more. Do you think that I'm too aggressive in my estimation of the level of perio in our patients?

Doctor Donut: No, not at all. I never thought of that. Why do you ask?

Heidi Hygienist: Well, there have been a few occasions where I have the patient totally aware of the degree of disease, and they're ready to make an appointment, and they leave with a lesson in brushing better.

Doctor Donut: Oh, I guess I do do that.

Heidi Hygienist: I'd also like to see parts of the schedule blocked, so that patients with periodontal disease can be seen sooner. Sometimes they have to wait for weeks to get an appointment.

Doctor Donut: That's easy enough to do with our system. Anything else?

Heidi Hygienist: I'd like to try those two things for three months, and then evaluate the progress instead of waiting another year. At the end of that three-month time, I'd like us to discuss the likelihood of having a dedicated dental hygiene assistant. I'm finding that I'm running behind because after I'm through talking to patients about treatment options, I still have to clean my room and take blood pressures and all the rest, when an assistant could be doing all of that and I could focus on patient care.

Doctor Donut: Wow, it looks like we need another one-hour discussion. I think I could be ready by Friday.

Heidi Hygienist: I look forward to it. I also have some ideas on creating a remineralization protocol. I'll bring in some literature.

Doctor Donut: You're just the kind of hygienist I've been looking for.

Heidi Hygienist: And you're an excellent clinician and artisan. Some of my hygiene friends are afraid of recommending cosmetic treatment at the offices they work in because of the poor results. I'm happy to be working here.

For some people this kind of dialog is nearly impossible. Maybe the boss is difficult, or maybe you

The Hard Raise

For my last review I was searching for a reason to show that I deserved a raise. Yes, I do produce, but mostly because it is a perio office and fees are high. I also take a lot of continuing education classes and try to introduce new things and ideas to the office. I take the time to tell the dentist about the things I learn and ask his opinion. I beg for new instruments and technology and back up my reasoning with good research. Bottom line, I put a lot of time into this office that is not actually "production" oriented, at least not in the short term.

So, for my closing remark at the review I left my boss with this thought: "I have worked here for over three years. In that period of time you have also had four other part-time hygienists join and leave the practice. There are only two hygienists who have ever stuck with you for more than three years - me and the Monday-Tuesday RDH, who has been here for five years. You have a reputation that precedes you, and many temps won't work for you based solely on that reputation. More than one hygienist has walked out in the middle of a day and never returned. So, equal in importance to the good I bring to this office is that fact that you can't afford to lose me. I have "put-up-with-you skills" that not many other hygienists in this area possess."

I not only got my raise, but the other RDH also got a raise in the middle of her review year. Use all of your assets.

— Lory (Lory is one of the hygienists participating in the Amyrdh e-mail community.)

lack confidence in yourself. We think this is so important that you should rehearse with someone, perhaps a hygienist friend that you trust. Don't do it with your husband or wife. That can get ugly. Do not bring up the salary of the other members of the team. If you compare yourself to the other hygienists in the office, you'll lose credibility points with your doctor. There is no way to compare yourself with others in the office without sounding jealous or petty.

Mentally prepare yourself with positive self-talk. If you're still having trouble, join Toastmasters International to get a handle on speaking for an audience. You'll gain the confidence you need to have a professional conversation like the one we have just outlined.

Keeping a Positive Attitude

In the chapter on networking, we discussed dealing with a sour hygienist, one who hates everything, one who is totally burned out. We wanted to tell you how we, and the people with whom we associate, maintain a positive attitude and prevent burnout.

Shirley never worked full-time in an office where she had an easy time. She stayed in the offices to maintain the income. She put up with a lot of grief, badgering, belittling, poor dentistry, and poor attitudes from other hygienists. She avoided them like the plague. She smiled and nodded, never argued with them, and made sure she wasn't like them. One of the ways Shirley kept herself from being just like them was to get a BSDH degree. She also discovered the Internet and found a group there that had the standards she wanted to live with.

Amy didn't have as strong a stomach as Shirley did. She found that the office was wrong for her right away, and kept looking until she found one that she really liked. Now she appreciates the dentist and he appreciates her. A win for all. What we had in common, and what we have in common with our friends who maintained a positive attitude about hygiene, is that we isolated ourselves from the negative people, and kept things around us new and fresh. We kept reading new things about dental hygiene. We tried new things with our patients, who really appreciated our efforts. We maintained a distance from the ordinary hygienist who chatted and polished and ignored disease.

Networking is one way to stay positive. It's easier to surround yourself with positive people if you have the means to get out of a small circle, like a practice setting. Another way is to try new things. Some things need permission from the practice owner, and some don't. Shirley had a lot of trouble recommending the water jet device in the last two offices where she worked. One doctor wanted to have the authority to decide what home care device his patients would benefit from. She kept recommending it because she knew it worked. It was a very difficult place to work, but she did it misguidedly, thinking she set a good example for her children, Actually, her frustration level was so high all the time that she couldn't even relate as a normal mom at home. Amy understood that and kept looking until something opened up where she could be comfortable at work.

Newness and freshness for hygienists is like garlic against vampires. Add a poster to your room. Try different instruments, read journals, and keep looking for the place that deserves you. Don't allow negativity to suck you dry. Hygiene careers can be very long and satisfying if you maintain mental and physical ergonomics.

Finally, to keep from becoming jaded, don't compromise. If the doctor continually asks you to practice in a way that is unethical according to your standards, or the broad standards of ethics established by our professional organization, or even the standards set by the dentist's organization, do yourself a favor and leave. Continually working at a level that is below your standards will leave you drained and conflicted. Eventually, you'll hate what you've become and that toxicity will flow over into your relationship with your patients, other staff members, and even your family.

Amy's first job was in an office where she fell in love with the beautiful reception room, not how good the equipment was or how competent the dentist was. She admired exactly what patients admire when they walk into a beautiful office. It was serene, it was clean, and it was orderly. It was designed to give patients a sense of comfort, and it worked on her.

The schedule was one patient every 45 minutes, which included taking any and all x-rays (including panorex and FMX), processing and mounting the films, perio charting, the prophy, and the exam! It was nearly impossible. At 32 years of age, Amy came home and cried every night. The schedule was intolerable. On days when she came home at 2 p.m., she would fall flat on the bed from exhaustion. Her kids would sit next to her on her bed watching TV as she lay passed out from a day's work as a dental hygienist. She was not just physically used up, but mentally as well. When she tried speaking to the dentist about her concerns at being so exhausted, he remarked, "Well, it took me ten years to become as great as I am, so maybe it will take you that long to get into a normal schedule, too." That was not a normal schedule.

The instruments at that office were horrible. A hand instrument broke in a patient's mouth once, and the ultrasonic scaler never worked. Meanwhile, the waiting room was the nicest she's ever seen. Amy was paid a certain set hourly wage. The practice had a bonus system where a production number was set, and if she averaged $100 an hour over that number for the week, she would get an extra $150 for that week. The dentist made it seem like it was an easy target. In reality, it was an impossible mark, and she never reached it. The x-rays she took weren't put down under her production; in addition, the office had a high rate of no-shows. The front desk blamed her for the high rate of open appointments. Amy, through her strong networking affiliations, was told by a previous hygienist that it had been that way when she worked there, too.

Amy only lasted five weeks at that office. She was depressed, crying daily, and feeling overwhelmed. She started to feel that she had made a bad decision by going into the dental hygiene profession.

With luck and the support of the Internet e-mail community, she looked for and immediately found another job in a wonderful office. She had an hour per patient, and there was a protocol for periodontal therapy which helped her understand how to treatment plan in the real world.

Her first office after her move to Nevada a few years later was a nightmare, too. It was not hygiene friendly at all. On any day, there were at least five hygienists working there. They were a great group, but it was an exceptionally toxic environment, in the figurative as well as the literal sense. It turned out that the section of the building in which the office was located had improper ventilation and the air was unhealthy. The whole staff was sick all the time. The monthly office meeting was full of negativity towards the hygiene department. The hygienists were always accused of doing everything wrong or not doing what others thought they should be doing. The entire department became burned out because of the negativity and their seclusion in their own part of the office. Amy lasted there an entire year. She was so miserable that she went so far as to get into arguments with the dentist purposefully, in hopes of getting fired. It just was not good.

After much trial and error in Nevada, Amy is now working with a highly competent dentist who does excellent work and is also a great person. The whole office gets along harmoniously. They help one another to make each day smoother. The patients notice that they all get along and remark about it all the time. Patients can tell they when the staff likes one another and there is an absence of tension in the office. Amy is allowed to make recommendations on patients' treatment plans when it comes to hygiene. She loves going to work and can tell that her work is better because she's not distracted by the stresses of a noxious environment and can truly appreciate what the office is doing for its patients every day.

Our advice to you is: Never stay in an office where you don't feel comfortable. There will always be glitches no matter where you work—no job is perfect—but look for an office where the quirks don't make you sick, or make you hate what you do. Ask yourself honestly if you are happy where you are. If you are constantly stressed, feel unappreciated, or if you feel like hygiene is not important in your office, it's a good idea to look elsewhere. Life is too short to spend time in venomous surroundings.

If you're reading this section and nodding your head, and have a tear in your eye because you see yourself here, you must be wondering how to find a job when you're not at your best. One thing to keep in mind is that the dental world is very small. We travel all around the country to the bigger dental meetings, and nearly always find someone there from our home state, if not our hometown. If the doctor you're working for has a poorly run office, everyone in town knows it. Drop off resumes, even if the office doesn't have an ad, keep friendly contact, and keep networking.

Bouncing Checks

What can you do if your paycheck bounces? No, don't go with your first gut reaction—you can't burn the dentist's house down. This is a very sticky situation. Know your rights before you do anything. Some states have very stringent rules against bouncing paychecks. Penalties for your employer can range from having a late fee assessed to having to triple your income, in which case it might be very much a benefit for you to have the check be late.

Call your state's labor department. This can be found in the phone book's government section, where the pages usually have a blue edge. Call and get the necessary information before you take any action. If the check bouncing is chronic, you'll need to find another job.

Insuring Yourself

Disability and malpractice insurance are two of the most underused security blankets in dental hygiene. Hygienists will purchase their own equipment, and pay for their own continuing education, but let the doctor's malpractice insurance umbrella cover them. They go blissfully along until suddenly a claim against the doctor's insurance prompts that insurance carrier to sue the unsuspecting hygienist for neglect or incompetence. It can happen, and it does happen. People who would never gamble overtly do so every single day when they practice without proper insurance coverage. The American Dental Hygienists' Association (www.adha.org) has malpractice insurance plans available

Fast Facts—

2,200 people will suffer a disabling injury every hour!

1 out of 88 homes will be damaged by fire.

1 out of 70 autos will be in a serious accident.

1 out of every 8 people will suffer a disability.

for members, and there are other plans available to purchase on your own.

There are also plans available privately or through the ADHA for disability insurance in the unlikely event of your injury. They cover not just injuries on the job, but injuries at home or at play as well. If you're walking to your car from the grocery store on an icy Thursday evening and slip and break your wrist, you're out of commission. Without disability insurance, you're also out of a paycheck for the duration of your recovery. If your wrist doesn't heal properly, you're sunk for another two months or longer. Disability insurance works like this: You pay premiums monthly or quarterly to cover a portion of your income. The larger the portion of your income you want to cover, the higher the premiums. Most plans will go into effect for pregnancy as well as injury or disability. Look into it, and then sit down and figure out if you are financially prepared to go without an income for six months. Or are you prepared to go without food on icy days, never play any sports, work in the garden, or even leave the house? Some larger practices offer long-term disability insurance as a benefit, or they offer a portion of the payment. Get it and have the premium deducted from your paycheck before you notice it.

9

FAQs

I am so nervous about going from three-hour appointments down to 45 or 60 minutes. I just don't know how I am going to do it. Can you offer any advice?

This book will help you with this transition. Ask your potential employer if you could have 60 minutes for at least the first few weeks so that you can adjust to working in real-world time constraints. Stay positive and know that it does get easier as we practice longer. Keep your chin up!

I don't know what the going rate for my area is. How can I find out?

You can always call your local ADHA component and ask them for advice on what the going rate is in your area. By networking with hygienists in your area, you can stay abreast of all the changes in going rates in your area. Another place to look is *RDH* magazine. Every year they put out a survey for hygienists to fill out and publish the results. Go to www.rdhmag.com and search for survey.

The new office that I work in does not have an ultrasonic scaler. I really want one to work with. What should I do?

Have you asked your new employer about an ultrasonic scaler? If not, try doing so. Explain that you will work more efficiently with it, not to mention the therapeutic benefits that the patient will receive. If your employer chooses to not get you one, you can either find a new position that better meets your needs or you can purchase your own.

By purchasing your own ultrasonic scaler, you can take it with you wherever you choose to work. In most cases, you will be able to deduct this expense from your income for tax purposes. The main thing is that you will be saving your own body.

Should I be carrying my own liability insurance?

Yes! You can get your own liability insurance for around $70-$90 a year. You should always be protected with your own coverage. In most cases, you will also be able to deduct this expense from your income. Look into disability insurance as well. This, of course, will be more of an expense than the liability insurance, but will be well worth it.

The new office I work in puts all new patients in my schedule. I am not comfortable with this. What should I do?

New patients should always see the doctor first. The doctor should diagnose any treatment that the patient needs. It also looks more professional to a patient that they are seeing the doctor first. If this is constantly happening in your office, you should talk to your dentist about this. If nothing is resolved, it might be a sign that you need to find another office. In most general supervision states, a hygienist can see a patient if a doctor is not present, but only if the patient is a patient of record. Make sure if you are seeing patients when the doctor isn't in that there are no new patients in your schedule.

I work in a large practice where much gossip goes on. How can I avoid getting involved in this without seeming rude?

It is much better to stay away from office gossip. You never know when it will come back to you. Don't be rude; when people start gossiping, you can simply say you need to get something done in your operatory or need to go over charts. Then make a clean exit. Be professional and don't get involved in that scene. If someone pursues you, explain that you don't engage in gossip. If necessary, you can even explain that it is a New Year's resolution or a religious conviction.

My office has a soft tissue management (STM) program. I have never heard of this—what is it?

STM is actually a registered trademark of the Prodentec company. It is their word for periodontal therapy, and many offices use that term. Just as the word Band-Aid is actually a brand name for a bandage, but people associate that term with all bandages and use the term interchangeably, STM is an all-encompassing term that refers to the protocol for treating periodontal disease.

Should I be using an ultrasonic scaler on demineralized areas?

No! This will cause the enamel to flake off and become weaker. Make sure you are practicing in-office and at-home remineralization protocols including fluorides, glass ionomers, Recaldent, xylitol, and chlorhexidine.

I want to send out a resume, however I live in a small dental community. I do not want my present boss to find out. How do I note it professionally that my inquiry is to be kept confidential?

When you send out a resume, make sure you state in your cover letter that you would like to keep your interest in a possible new position confidential from your present employer.

I am going to school in one state but want to move to another. How do I know if I need to take another clinical board?

You will need to check with each individual state to find out what their requirements are for licensure. Many states that participate in a regional board like the NERB will accept your clinical exam. You may have to take a jurisprudence exam for the new state you intend to move to. There are a few states that comprise their own board. Some states require that you retake your national boards if they have not been taken within a certain amount of time. If you ever think you may move at some point, it is good to check these things out ahead of time. With good prior planning, you may be able to avoid the expense and hassle of retaking the boards.

My office wants me to give all adults a fluoride treatment. I don't feel it's necessary. What should I do?

Most adults will benefit greatly from a fluoride treatment. Not just in-office, but at-home fluorides as well. It is great that your office advocates fluoride for adults. Many offices do not, since insurance won't cover it. The bottom line is that the doctor has the final say and you are obliged to follow his or her orders.

Since I just graduated in May, do I need CEs for the upcoming renewal this December?

Check with your state board. Every state is different. Part of your licensure is to keep abreast of all the changes to regulations that affect dental hygiene practice. You can contact your state board. Many states have required courses that you need to take. Check into the limitations on the number of courses that you can take at home or online.

I have received two job offers. One is close to home, but that office is not offering me as much money as the one farther from home. I do get a better feeling about the office close to home, but I want to make the higher salary. What should I do?

Weigh all your options, but do not let money make your choices for you. Really think about this. Money will not make you happy in toxic situations. You will burn out fast if you are only choosing due to pay scale. Sometimes toxic, stressful offices have to offer more money just to get someone to work there. Those offices usually have a high turnover rate. Figure out how much it will cost you to drive every day. Figure in gas and also call your auto insurance company. It may make the closer office a bargain!

10

Meet the Authors

Shirley Gutkowski received her associate's degree in dental hygiene in 1986, after which she started full-time clinical practice working for a temporary agency. After two years, she began working in Madison, WI for a single dentist, forty hours per week. Shirley maintained that level of practice until 1995, when she allowed herself to cut out one day per week.

She and her husband have five sons, and after the children were grown, she returned to school and earned a baccalaureate degree in dental hygiene, graduating in 1999. She regularly takes part in a number of dental and non-dental Internet group discussions, which give her a unique perspective on all of dentistry, including dentists, hygienists, other staff positions, and most importantly, patients.

Shirley began writing a monthly column in *RDH* magazine in 2001 and writes feature articles for that magazine as well as other dental periodicals and consumer publications. In the summer of 2003, her speaking and writing career had begun to take so much time that she was no longer able to provide clinical care for patients.

As a child, Shirley really wanted to be a teacher and or an actress. Dental hygiene ended up fitting that bill nicely. All day she taught people a special skill, and she had a new audience every hour, laughing at the same five jokes for a six-month run. Continuing education is a high priority for her, and she attends continuing education courses three or four times a year, incorporating something from each course into her daily routine.

Amy Nieves attended college to study accounting after she graduated from high school. After a year she dropped out, because the subject matter wasn't stimulating enough for her. She could never imagine sitting at a desk and doing someone's taxes over and over again. She started taking a few classes at the local community college in 1994, thinking she'd like to be a teacher. At that time in New Jersey, however, there were few teaching jobs and she was told by a friend that it was "not *what* you know but *who* you know that gets you a job."

With this specter over her head, she started to rethink her interests. Amy was taking a science course and learned about the dental hygiene profession. With her interest aroused, she looked into it. She pursued the prerequisites and was accepted into the program.

Amy graduated with an associate's degree in dental hygiene in 1999. Today she is the moderator of one of the most important dental hygiene e-mail communities on the Internet. She moderates an e-mail community for students, keeping abreast of all the problems plaguing them as they enter our special world and the RDH e-mail community for practicing hygienists. The RDH list is comprised of all types of dental hygienists the world over, including clinical hygienists, corporate hygienists, entrepreneur hygienists, and every kind in between, as well as a few special dentists.

In the short time she has been a hygienist, Amy has seen both the good and bad sides of the profession. Today she's in "hygiene heaven" and loving every moment of her career. She has attended over 40 CE hours yearly since graduating. Amy thinks of herself as a sponge that just wants to soak up every amount of knowledge possible. In addition to her career as a dental hygienist, Amy is a busy wife and the mother of three children.

Index

antibiotic, 31, 32, 45, 58, 79, 81-85, 88, 102, 106, 124
ADHA, 9, 13, 65-66, 129, 137, 139
anesthetic, 23, 84, 87, 100, 102-103, 109-110, 117
Arestin, 58, 106, 124
Atridox, 58, 106, 124
bleach, 38, 46, 52, 64, 104, 115, 121, 128
blood pressure, 43, 55, 83, 90, 93, 124, 131
burnout, 41, 51, 132
comission, 23-24, 33-34, 125-126, 137
cytology, 63
D0120, 61, 63
D0150, 61
D0180, 61
D0350, 61
D0415, 62
D0425, 62
D1110, 62, 103-104
D1310, 62

D1320, 62
D1330, 61, 62, 107
D1351, 62, 107
D2940, 62
D2970, 62
D4341, 63, 101, 103
D4342, 63
D4355, 63
D4381, 63, 101, 106
D4910, 63, 103-104
D5986, 63
D7286, 63
D9215, 64, 101, 102
D9910, 64, 110
D9911, 64
D9920, 64
D9972, 64
dry mouth, 124
Fast Fact, 19, 40, 52, 60, 62, 76, 81, 102, 124, 137
glass ionomer, 60, 64, 107, 141
home care, 57, 102-103, 133

instruments, 25, 55, 58, 76, 77, 78, 100, 101, 105, 113, 109, 125
insurance, x, 37-43, 48, 61-62, 92, 104, 118, 124, 129, 136-137, 140, 142
morning huddle, 29, 56-57
networking, 65, 72, 77, 132-134, 136, 139
periodontal, 4, 6-8, 10, 23, 29, 32, 39, 40, 45-46, 49, 51-53, 57-59, 61, 63, 80, 84, 86-87, 90, 92-93, 96, 100, 102-105, 116, 124, 127-128, 130, 134, 141
periodontal therapy, 7, 10, 29, 32, 39, 40, 51, 57, 58, 59, 61, 63, 80, 86, 90, 93, 102, 103, 104, 105, 124, 134, 141